PAIN

It's Not All in Your Head

The Tests Don't Show Everything

Jay Tracy PA-C, Psy.D., L.P.

National Library of Canada Cataloguing in Publication

Tracy, Jay, 1950-
  It's not all in your head : the tests don't show everything / Jay Tracy ; Geoff Daily, illustrator.

ISBN 1-55369-415-5

1. Self-care, Health. I. Title.

RC81.T72 2002   616.02'4   C2002-901674-6

TRAFFORD

This book was published on-demand in cooperation with Trafford Publishing.
On-demand publishing is a unique process and service of making a book available for retail sale to the public taking advantage of on-demand manufacturing and Internet marketing.
On-demand publishing includes promotions, retail sales, manufacturing, order fulfilment, accounting and collecting royalties on behalf of the author.

Suite 6E, 2333 Government St., Victoria, B.C. V8T 4P4, CANADA
Phone   250-383-6864   Toll-free   1-888-232-4444 (Canada & US)
Fax   250-383-6804   E-mail   sales@trafford.com
Web site   www.trafford.com   TRAFFORD PUBLISHING IS A DIVISION OF TRAFFORD HOLDINGS LTD.
Trafford Catalogue #02-0228   www.trafford.com/robots/02-0228.html

10   9   8   7   6   5   4   3

From the staff at the Chronic Pain Rehabilitation Program, Sister Kenny Institute, Abbott Northwestern Hospital, Minneapolis, Minnesota:

"Dr. Tracy has written a very thorough overview of the pain experience capturing all of the variants and complexities in a very succinct and engaging manner. Although the language is directed to the individual with pain, this is an excellent resource for anyone interested in the subject. It was a great, fun, funny effective and quick read. It's the explanations and metaphors that would help other professionals understand and explain the muddied waters. Nice job."

Peg Kellar, RN, CNS
Clinical Nurse Specialist

"The experience of pain is universal. Over the centuries healers of diverse cultures have discovered a plethora of techniques for treating pain. These practices vary from the very ancient such as acupuncture and herbs to the very modern interventional approaches of injections, new pharmacologic agents, surgery, and the use of implantable devices directly into the central nervous system. Despite the implementation of these techniques, low tech and high tech, interventional and alternative, ancient and modern, satisfactory resolution of the experience of pain for many remains elusive. It has been estimated that as many as 25 million Americans experience some form of chronic pain.
Individuals experiencing pain, particularly chronic pain often seek treatment from multiple clinicians. They spend hundreds of hours and they and their insurance companies spend thousands, and sometimes hundreds of thousands of dollars searching for the "cure". These individuals are often given multiple diagnoses, undergo numerous diagnostic and therapeutic interventions, and when all is said and done continue to have

pain as their constant companion. Their experience with the health care system is frequently disappointing in the least, and at the extreme, downright disastrous.

With this book, Dr. Tracy has made an heroic effort to "get his hands around" an incredibly complex subject and present this information in a clear, concise manner, that is easily understandable. Starting with an explanation of the theories, and the accepted pathophysiology of many painful conditions, he nicely progresses into a discussion of accepted treatment options. He ends his book with his perspective of nearly 30 years, as a physician's assistant, psychologist, and above all as a compassionate human being, communicating clearly the importance of both the physical as well as psychosocial and spiritual perspectives required in understanding the complexities and treatment options in addressing chronic pain.

All individuals experiencing chronic pain, their families, and health professionals who interact with them should read this book. By both simplifying difficult concepts and clarifying why these ambiguities exist, Dr. Tracy's work is an excellent primer for those interested in this subject."

Mathew Monsein, MD
Medical Director

"Among the most pressing of needs for a person with ongoing pain is the need of understandable information regarding his or her medical condition, as well as the need for validation that the pain is real. Dr. Tracy meets both in this landmark text. He is able to reduce complex medical terminology to understandable terms and interweave experiences and emotions to make this a compelling and interesting read. He also validates the individual's experience given a medical condition that is virtually unseen by others.

Dr. Tracy brings his almost 30 years of experience to the forefront in this text. He describes normal anatomy and physiolo-

gy and then details what can happen to cause pain. What then sets this book apart from other writings is his excellent description of the pain experience and how this can affect all areas of a person's life. He leaves the reader with hope by answering a series of most commonly asked questions.

Remarkably comprehensive and informative, this book is a must not only for individuals with pain, but for their support system and for any professionals working with these individuals."

Nancy Carlson, Psy.D., L.P.
Director of Psychological Services

Preface

You've been injured in a car accident or on the job. You are continuing to experience neck pain and associated headaches. You are worried about symptoms of numbness, tingling, weakness and pain in your arms and fingers. You are experiencing low back pain with radiation into your buttocks, legs and feet. You've seen a doctor or several doctors. You've had some tests that have come back "normal". You've tried several treatment approaches but have only experienced temporary relief. You are having difficulties keeping up at work. You have cut down on certain activities at home, with friends, or for enjoyment. You don't know what to do or where to go from here. You are irritable, frustrated, afraid and worried about the future. You wonder if you're going crazy and if others think "the problem is all in your head".

DO NOT DESPAIR! THERE IS HOPE! YOU ARE NOT ALONE! THERE ARE MANY THINGS THAT CAN BE DONE. THERE ARE MANY ISSUES THAT NEED TO BE ADDRESSED.

First of all, you're not crazy. You are a normal person. The sources of the pain are not "all in your head." They are usually in the body. Medical tests and technology still do not show everything. If the doctor says, "Your test is normal," just remember that *the tests don't show everything*.

However, you are responsible for what is in your head. What is in your head affects how you recover. Information helps. No information confuses. Options help. No options make you feel trapped, imprisoned, tense and tight in your own muscles, thoughts, feelings, and lifestyle.

Acknowledgements and special thanks to:

Lawrence J. Schut, MD, for many years of friendship and training in helping people control and deal better with chronic neurologic diseases, disabilities, and abilities. I thank him for teaching me the importance of seeking the correct diagnosis and establishing the treatment plan in cooperation with the patient and family. I also thank him for helping me to understand that the "optimum level of functioning" (OLOF) is really a compromise between the patient's perspective and that of the professionals involved.

Alfred V. Anderson, DC, MD., much of the information, format, and ideas with respect to the psychophysiologic profile come from his education of patients.

Ralph E. McKinney, Ph.D., L.P., my friend and mentor, who continues to teach me, by his life and example, how to really care for the people, and how to give them power in creative, enjoyable and meaningful ways.

Steve Harr, PA-C, for his friendship and work in the pain management program in the past, and for his well written ideas and review of myofascial pain.

The Minneapolis Clinic of Neurology, Ltd., its doctors, staff, and my friends in the Rehabilitation Associates Pain Management Program, for all their support in helping patients with pain.

The staff of the Pain Management Program at Sister Kenny Institute at Abbott Northwestern Hospital for the training and insights into chronic pain and various treatment approaches. For caring, normalization, validation, and motivation for change.

My daughter, *Megan*, for her computer skills and graphic designs.

My friend, *Geoff Daily*, for his technical editing and desktop publishing skills, his creative artistic work, and his willingness to try new things and work beyond the simple approaches.

My patients and their families for all of their work and contributions in improving their own and each others very difficult situations.

Table of Contents

Introduction

The medical approach to pain has two parts: **Diagnosis** and **Treatment**.

Diagnosis:

Essential to effective pain treatment is diagnosis--why are you in pain? What is causing the pain? The medical professionals need to clarify the diagnosis in their own minds and then share that information with you in as much detail as possible. Your understanding of what's going on with your body will help to ensure a successful treatment plan. Sometimes a clear-cut diagnosis is not possible. This happens. It may not matter where you go, who you saw, or what tests are done. The doctor may not really know exactly what is going on. In those cases it is important that all other likely causes of pain have been evaluated and excluded. It is important in those cases also that a doctor that you trust explains to you as best he or she can what they think is going on.

The diagnosis is made on the basis of your history and physical examination coupled with diagnostic testing. In most cases, this combined approach provides the needed answers to proceed with appropriate treatment. Even though the results of diagnostic tests come back normal, this does not mean that there isn't a physical reason for the pain. **Tests don't show everything**. Each diagnostic procedure is performed specifically to evaluate certain anatomical, chemical or physiological functions to determine the cause of the pain. For example, simple x-rays mainly show bones. The CT (computerized tomographic) scan shows both bone and soft tissue, but not completely. A myelogram is another anatomical test which provides a different perspective of back and neck problems but it still does not reveal everything. The same is true of the MRI (magnetic resonance imaging), which shows significant anatomical detail. Electromyography (EMG) and thermography show the function of nerves but can also come back "normal" even in the face of severe pain. Normal test results do not mean that you are not in pain or that the problem is imaginary. Normal tests indicate that certain, specific causes for the pain, only specific things that the specific test is looking for, were not found to be present. To repeat, normal tests do not mean that you don't have pain. Many people sometimes forget this simple but important point.

Understanding your diagnosis is very important. Do you know what your diagnosis is? Can you explain it to someone else clearly and accurately? Do you feel comfortable and confident at least that the diagnosis is right or as close to right as possible? Do you feel fairly confident that nothing is being missed?

If the answers are yes, you have a good foundation for improvement in your situation. If the answers are no, then it is going to be even more difficult for you to understand your treatment and what to expect for the future concerning this ongoing pain problem.

You might ask, can't the doctor just know what is going on and tell me the treatment plan and prognosis for the future? Yes and no. If yours is a relatively simple pain problem, yes. But if it is a more complicated situation where pain is ongoing, it may be difficult for anyone to make the diagnosis very clear. Further, it may be very difficult to establish a good treatment plan and accurate prognosis.

If the basis for the pain is not easily understood or solved, you are the person who has to manage and deal with this pain problem, your pain problem. However, this doesn't have to be done alone. Your doctor and your team of professionals and your support system can help you. But you have to be in charge of your team much as you can.

Understanding your diagnosis as much as possible can help. Understanding and information will help lessen some of the fear of the unknown. Fear may not be the cause of the pain, but fear, uncertainty, and lack of knowledge can increase or worsen pain perception. Fear may also worsen your physical and emotional responses to pain. Fear may make muscles tighter, cause ulcers, increased blood pressure, sweating, numbness and odd sensations into the extremities. Underlying fear may make you more irritable, frustrated, depressed, angry. You may feel worried, anxious, guilty, and tend to blame yourself or others for the many problems associated with stress. Ignorance isn't always bliss.

Treatment:

After a diagnosis has been established, the next step is to consider a treatment program. In cases of neck and back pain, this means either an operation or no operation. That is, the pain is treated either with: 1. surgery, or 2. conservative treatment.

1. Surgery

Surgery is usually not the first step, but it is often a treatment consideration. While we may try different forms of conservative treatment, surgery might be the only approach that can really fix the problem. When you take your car to the shop to be fixed, the mechanic listens to your story, examines the car when opening the hood (diagnosis), takes something out, adjusts something, puts something back in (treatment), closes the hood and he is finished (don't we wish?). The car is fixed - surgically. But you are not a car. We cannot "open the hood" and dig around inside to figure out what is wrong and fix it. This type of "exploratory surgery" used to be done in the past more often, but was not usually very successful, and often worsened the problems rather than helped. The point is, surgery is usually done for a quite specific purpose based upon the diagnostic information.

Surgical treatment is recommended for one of two reasons. One, you are hurting "bad enough" that you come to the doctor after unsuccessful conservative treatment and say, "I'm hurting so bad now, something has to be done! Cut my arm off, cut my head off, shoot me, I don't care, but do something!" This is fairly extreme but it might be the way you feel sometimes. If feeling this badly is diminished by conservative treatment and you are left with lesser routine daily pain, then neck or back surgery could (and usually should) be avoided. The risks of surgery always need to be weighed against its potential benefit.

The second reason to do surgery is progressive nerve damage. Progressive nerve injury may not be the same as feeling worse with pain and associated symptoms. You may be feeling pain but the nerves still work well. The nerves can be "irritated" or "rubbed on" yet function properly. We determine evidence of nerve damage by the physical examination--checking reflexes, muscles, sensation and by using other tests such as EMG or thermography to measure the function of nerves and compare one time to another time. If a nerve is showing progressive damage as evidenced by the exam findings or test results, then surgery might be appropriate. If the risks of not doing surgery outweigh the risks of doing surgery, then surgery might be done.

2. Conservative treatment

"Conservative" means "not surgery." Conservative treatment is usually tried first before considering surgery, for many times relatively simple measures can provide adequate relief. Conservative treatment methods are divided into passive and active forms.

Passive conservative is something done to you. All you have to do is receive it. These forms of treatment include physical therapy (like heat, massage, ultrasound, traction, and many other passive forms of physical therapy), medications, TENS (transcutaneous electrical nerve stimulator), whirlpool, acupuncture, acupressure, manipulation or gentle mobilization, cervical pillow, cervical collar. The goal of these techniques is to promote healing in the acute phase of an injury. Also, they can help you get through significant, acute flare-ups, which often occur when struggling with chronic pain. In the long run, if you are dealing with a long-term problem, you need a treatment approach that will give you long term benefits. When the pain problem is past the healing phase, you may need more than passive conservative treatment alone. There are forms of physical therapy called myofascial trigger point release techniques or other manual techniques that utilize both passive and active approaches and thereby promote more long term benefits rather than simply temporary relief.

Active conservative is something that you do yourself. This approach may have more potential for long term relief and benefit. Your body begins healing from the second you are hurt. It is important not to impair the healing process by doing non-healthy things. These include but are not limited to smoking, drinking alcohol too much, using drugs inappropriately, eating poorly, using too much caffeine, not sleeping adequately, not exercising, continuing to abuse your body by overdoing, re-injuring yourself, not pacing yourself in your activities, taking care of everybody else instead of taking care of yourself, and poor stress and conflict management. These are all complex issues and involve your personality, your habits, goals, your desires, and all the demands of the situation you are in. Not everything is under your complete control. However, you will need to take the active role in changing what you can to make the difference between healing as well as you can and not healing well. Some specific things you can do are as follows.

Specific body part exercises for neck or back can promote improved range of motion, stretching, flexibility, relaxation, strengthening. These exercises can be done in combination with some of the passive conservative approaches. Many of the active conservative treatment approaches can be used in combination with the passive conservative approaches very successfully. General body endurance building may increase endorphins, your own body's pain-killing chemicals. Exercise can help vent frustration, help prevent flare-ups or at least lessen the frequency, duration and possibly even the severity of acute flare-ups. Relaxation techniques, mental imagery, self-hypnosis, other stress management techniques can all be helpful and are active in that you have to do them yourself. Learning as much as you can about your diagnosis, treatment options, and expectations for the future can also be very helpful in the long run.

You might be struggling with the idea that you might have to accept this pain problem. This is hard. This does not mean "giving up" or "giving up hope." You may need a compassionate, loving, treatment approach. You may need to deal with the grief process, denial, anger, depression, bargaining, acceptance -- a constantly up and down, moving and dynamic experience. All these approaches are active yet conservative.

To Get The Most Out Of This Book:

Studies show that one of the most important determining factors for college students to do well is whether or not they show up for class. They will do even better if they sit in front and ask questions and are really involved as opposed to sitting in back and twiddling their thumbs. They will do even better if they do the homework.

The same applies in lessening and dealing with pain. This particular workbook requires that you ask and answer questions. Work slowly and carefully. It can make a great difference for you and the people important to you.

Formulate specific questions about your own diagnosis, treatment options, expectations for the future, and the effects on your life. Write them all down. Ask the people close to you, your spouse, your family members, friends, employer, fellow employees, etc. as appropriate to write down their own questions about the whole situation.

Write down your own answers to the various questions that have been asked. Then read the book, a little at a time. Underline or mark the parts that apply to you.

Share the questions, answers and readings of this book with the people close to you as appropriate. You may be surprised at how much others want to care or be helpful. But often others don't know what to do or say and many times will do or say things that are very hurtful.

It will help you to understand your own situation very clearly first. Then you can help others to understand better as well, if they really want to. If you are dealing with someone who truly doesn't care, then don't waste too much energy on them. And don't give them too much power over you. You have enough work to do just to gain further control of yourself and your pain situation.

Commonly Asked Questions:

Q. *Do you know what's really wrong in your back, neck or wherever the pain is?*

Q. *Do you understand why pain can last so long?*

Q. *Do you understand why the tests you've had are normal or at least may not be showing the problem clearly?*

Q. *Do you understand why further tests might not be of help?*

Q. *Do you understand what can and cannot be done about the pain to lessen it or make it go away?*

Q. *Do you know what to expect for the future?*

Q. *Does your doctor want to know your opinion about what the problem is?*

Q. *Does your doctor seem to give a short, simple, explanation for your medical problem, such as, "It's all in your head," or "It's just due to stress, age, height, weight?"*

Q. *Does your spouse, or anyone else in particular, look at things in a similar way, stating something like, "All you need is to get off your medicines" or "All you need is psychotherapy to deal with your personality disorder?"*

Q. *Do you know what your limitations are for safety and comfort, or if you really have any limitations, or how long they will last?*

Q. *Do you know how to live well or happily in spite of the pain that is remaining?*

Q. *Are you sure the injured person is not faking?*

Q. *If he can go to a play or do some other recreational activity, why can't he work more hours? If the person can ride a motorcycle, why can't he work?*

Q. *How long does it take for things to heal? They said it would just take time but this has already been a long time.*

Q. *Why can't they just fix this problem?*

Q. *I've been to several doctors. One tells me this, another tells me that. They can't agree and I am in between.*

Q. *It seems that the insurance company is only out to save dollars. They don't care about me. They just force me back to work and don't care if it hurts.*

Q. *If it hurts, I am not going to do it. Pain has a purpose and it is telling me this isn't safe. At least, I don't want to be so flared-up that I can't enjoy anything after doing a particular activity.*

Q. *I can't accept that this problem is going to be permanent.*

Q. *I am beginning to wonder myself if the problem isn't imaginary.*

Q. *If I just didn't have this pain or if they could just fix the pain problem, I wouldn't have all these other emotional, financial, relationship, vocational and recreational problems.*

Q. *This person isn't doing the work he used to do, but I think he could, really, if he wanted to. Look at the professional football quarterback who had back surgery and went back to playing professional football.*

Q. *I am not depressed, I am just tired all the time. I don't feel like doing anything. I have no energy, no zip. I don't know what is wrong with me.*

Q. *Why shouldn't I use pain pills? They are the only things that help. They keep me going. They make me able to keep up some normal activities.*

Q. *If exercise makes things hurt worse, I am not going to do it. Is it really a matter of "no pain no gain"?*

Q. *What are discs?*

Q. *What are they made of and what do they do?*

Q. *What is a "bulging" or "herniated" disc, and which is worse?*

Q. *What is "degenerated" or "deteriorated" or "dehydrated"?*

Q. *Are discs strong?*

Q. *Can a bulging disc become a herniated disc?*

Q. *What can X-rays show?*

Q. *My CT scan or MRI showed a deteriorated and bulging disc, but my doctor said this was "normal". How can this be "normal"? I'm hurting like crazy?*

Q. *What is "spurring"? And what about "arthritis"?*

Q. *Can scar tissue form, and can it be helpful or harmful?*

Q. *Can a disc go back to its normal shape given enough time, and can a disc heal in the wrong shape and still cause pain?*

Q. *Sometimes the pain goes away or lessens for a while, but then comes back again. Why is this?*

Q. *Can they replace the inside of the disc with something else?*

Q. *Can they operate on the same disc more than once?*

Q. *I don't want to know about this stuff. I just want it fixed so I can go back to work again.*

Q. *Why don't they just do a CT scan or better yet an MRI and just find out what the problem is and fix it?*

Q. *What do they mean by soft tissue injury, myofascial pain, muscle ligament strain?*

Q. *Are they sure something isn't being missed? I mean I hurt soft tissue and pulled muscles before but that pain went away in a few days or weeks. This pain isn't going away.*

Q. *What is carpal tunnel syndrome? What can I expect for the future?*

Q. What is thoracic outlet syndrome? What can I expect for the future?

Q. What is fibromyalgia? What can I expect for the future?

Q. What is mechanical back pain? What are facet joints?

Q. What is reflex sympathetic dystrophy? What can I expect for the future? Will I damage anything if I use the limb too much? What is too much?

Q. What about diet and pain control?

Q. How can exercise help my problems?

Q. What are trigger points? Why would I want to have injections in these areas that are sore? Why does one doctor suggest these and another doesn't?

Notes:

Chapter 1: NORMAL ANATOMY AND PHYSIOLOGY

Bones (vertebrae)

Joints

Discs

Ligaments

Tendons

Muscles

Fascia

Nerves

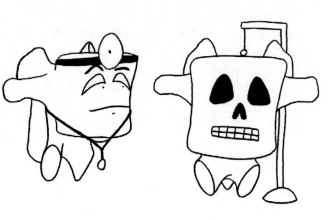

The neck and back can hurt. You know that already. But you may not know what specifically is injured, why it hurts, or how each type of pain can mean specific types of problems. Part of lessening or dealing with pain is understanding why you hurt. The back and neck are pretty complicated regions with each part causing specific types of pain. So, let's first see how they are put together.

There are supporting and other structures that work together to hold us upright as well as to move and bend our body with ease. These parts are constantly fighting the downward pull of gravity. Back pain is the price that we have paid in the evolution from a four-legged to two-legged posture as the whole body weight focuses in the back. We'll talk about weight loss later. The neck is also subjected to these gravitational forces as it works to hold up the 10-15 pound head, about the weight of a bowling ball. The supporting and other structures are: bones (vertebrae), joints, discs, ligaments, tendons, fascia, muscles, and nerves.

Bones (vertebrae)

The vertebrae are individual bones stacked upon each other like blocks to form the vertebral column or "back bone." (Vertebra = one bone, singular. Vertebrae = more than one bone, plural.) It is only because of the back bone that we are able to stand straight and tall - leaving personality considerations aside. The vertebral column is subdivided into five different regions:

1) the cervical region is the neck with the skull on top,
2) the thoracic region is through the length of the trunk,
3) the lumbar region is the low back area,
4) the sacral region is just below that and
5) the coccyx makes up the "tail bone."

A specific number of vertebrae are associated with each region: The cervical has 7 vertebrae. Did you know that both humans and giraffes have the same number of vertebrae in the neck - 7? The thoracic region has 12 vertebrae. The lumbar has 5. The sacrum is actually 4 or 5 vertebrae which become fused by 25 years of age. The coccyx is also a fused vertebra in adults. We need to know these numbers because the vertebrae are named according to their level. For example, the sixth vertebra in the cervical (neck) region is the C6 (cervical - 6) vertebra; the fifth vertebra in the thoracic region is T5 (thoracic - 5); the fourth vertebra in the lumbar region is the L4 (lumbar - 4) vertebra; and so on.

The spaces between the vertebrae are also named, quite simply, according to the vertebrae above and below that space. For example, the L5-S1 space is between the fifth lumbar (L5) vertebra and the sacrum (S1). So, if your doctor says that you have an L4-L5 disc herniation, this means the disc is out between the L4 and L5 vertebrae. We'll talk about disc herniation later.

At birth, the vertebral column is straight. As we start walking, the force of gravity acts upon this upright posture and two gentle curves develop in the vertebral

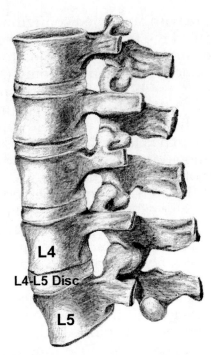

column. The cervical curve forms in the neck region at about 3 months of age when we start holding our heads up. The lumbar curve forms in the low back area by the end of our first year of life when we start standing. The combined effect of these curves is to produce a roughly S-shape in the vertebral column. These curves are easily seen on x-rays. To the novice looking at cervical and lumbar x-rays, these curvatures may appear abnormal like something is "out of line." But, they are very normal.

The shapes of the vertebrae from each level are different. This is because the vertebrae from the different levels are subjected to different types of stresses and muscular forces. Regardless of their shape, most vertebrae have the same parts. In front is a large cylindrical portion termed the body which is the weight-bearing portion of the vertebra. Since the lumbar vertebrae in the low back region carry the weight from the upper half of the torso, the bodies of these vertebrae are the largest of the vertebrae. Sticking out from the back of the vertebra is a more delicate structure with an arched configuration. A portion of the arch is called the lamina. When surgery for discs is performed, the surgeon cuts the lamina to get to the disc in a procedure known as a laminectomy (ectomy = to cut away). Since only the body of the vertebra is the weight bearing portion, cutting the lamina part of the vertebra has no effect on the vertebra's ability to support the torso. At the top of the arch is the spinous process or spine. You can feel the spinous processes in the middle of your own back as a series of bumps aligned in a row. An open area in the center of the arch is termed the vertebral foramen. When the vertebra are aligned in a row, the vertebral foramen of each vertebra together form a tunnel, the vertebral canal. This effect is like stacking a number of napkin rings. Look down the center of this stack and you have made a vertebral canal. The vertebral canal contains and protects the spinal cord and nerve roots down to the L1 vertebra. Past that level, this space only contains nerve fibers or wires, not a solid spinal cord.

The vertebrae hurt because they are covered by a thin membrane called periosteum which is highly pain-sensitive. A fracture or injury to the bone causes irritation of the periosteum resulting in significant pain.

Joints

Joints are the way that one bone is connected to another bone. Joints allow movement between those bones. If it weren't for joints, we would be stiff, solid beings incapable of any movement. The vertebrae connect with one another by joints, termed facets. The facets allow movement in both front-to-back and side-to-side directions. Each vertebra has four facets. Two facets pivot on the vertebra sitting on top and two facets pivot on the vertebra below. The facets provide flexibility of movement for the vertebral column, permitting us to bend in all directions. Like all joints of the body such as the shoulders and knuckles, the facets are lined with tissue and surrounded by a thin capsule of ligament tissue

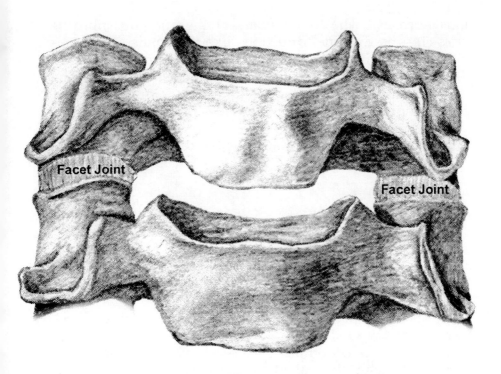

which is pain sensitive. And, like all joints, the facets may become irritated and painful producing spine pain.

The sacroiliac joint is another type of joint in the low back area. The sacrum is a long vertebra, or a series of 4 or 5 vertebrae which fuse by adulthood. The sacrum connects the vertebral column to the pelvis. The joint between the sacrum and the hip or pelvic bones (iliac bones) is the sacroiliac joint. This area is also a pain sensitive region.

Discs

Discs are hockey puck-shaped cushions located in the spaces between the vertebrae. For example, the C5-C6 disc is located between the fifth and sixth cervical vertebrae. Pretty logical, huh?

Structurally, each disc has a firm, fibrous outside layer and a jelly-like inner core. The outer layer is called the annulous fibrosus. The tough fibers of the annulous fibrosus criss-cross in diagonal directions like the bands on a steel-belted radial tire. This arrangement gives the disc strength. The inner core of the disc is called the nucleus pulposus. The nucleus pulposus, made of gelatinous protein, is contained by the annulous fibrosus and provides the cushion effect.

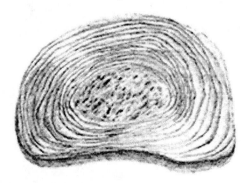

The outside can wear out over time, or can tear suddenly in an injury. Then the inside can push or ooze through to the outside, like toothpaste out of a toothpaste tube. If this occurs, it might be called a "herniated", "ruptured", or "slipped" disc. A "bulging" disc might be the same thing only less severe. It might be that the inside is not all the way through to the outside. Damage to the outside of the disc or tearing of the outside of the disc can cause weakening of the fibrous bands resulting in a "bulging" disc. If the fibers are torn severely, the inner gelatinous core may extrude out through the annulous fibrosus, resulting in a herniated disc.

Think of a disc like a bismark donut. The jelly-like substance can ooze through to the outside and press against the nerve next to it, sending symptoms into an arm or leg or anyplace in the body where the nerve goes.

Discs are very strong. If we squeezed straight up and down on the column of bones and discs hard enough, the bones would crack and crumble before the discs gave way. However, if we squeeze with more of a slant, or wedging, the discs may "pop" or rupture. Twisting movements are also very hard on them and can result in a tearing, shearing, or wearing out of the outside and a bulging through of the inside.

Think of the disc as a grape. If you squeeze a grape a little bit, it tends to bulge in the middle, as would a bulging disc. However, if you keeping applying pressure, the grape will eventually "pop." The grape covering tears and the inside of the grape shoots out, resulting in a "ruptured" or "herniated" grape. A herniated disc occurs in a similar fashion. A "contained disc" might be like the bulging grape, whereas a "non-contained disc" might be like the herniated or ruptured grape.

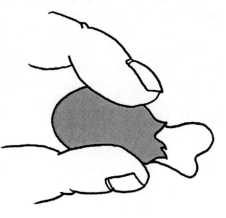

If a grape (like a disc) sits on a shelf a long time and doesn't move at all, it tends to dry up, turning into a raisin. This might be thought of as a degenerated or deteriorated disc. We all get some of this as we grow older. From the age of twenty to eighty we might lose two to six inches in height due to disc narrowing, wearing out, flattening, or drying up. This usually doesn't cause any symptoms, but certainly can cause problems if the nerves near the disc are irritated. Actually, on a percentage basis, disc disease may account for only a small portion of pain from the spine, particularly chronic pain.

We can see vertebrae but not discs on simple x-rays of the back or neck. The x-rays go right through a disc. Discs can be seen by CT or MRI scanning. But even on these effective tests the disc pathology might not show up clearly. If a disc is worn out or herniated, that disc space may be narrowed because of the lessened volume of the nucleus pulposus. So, if we see a narrow disc space on regular x-rays, this finding may suggest significant disc disease at that level. However, bulging and narrowed discs can be seen in people who have no symptoms at all. Therefore, the physician has to put the whole story together, the history, the examination findings, and the test results. He or she then has to give an opinion about what really might be going on.

The body may form calcium, bone spurring, all around the edges of the bones above and below the disc in an attempt to hold the disc still and to protect it. Scar tissue may form around a herniated or bulging disc to help strengthen and support the disc.

The discs can still be strong after they have been injured. The outside of the disc, the annulous fibrosus, does have a blood supply, but not very much. Therefore, it may not heal quickly after an injury, but often a disc can recover and become healthy and strong. The toothpaste can go back into the toothpaste tube if it wasn't out very far in the first place.

After surgery to remove a disc, the body may form fibrous, hard, calcified scar tissue inside and around the operated part of the disc. The disc space can narrow after surgery and result in facet problems, nerve irritation, and continued symptoms in a limb.

Ligaments

Ligaments are fibrous, elastic bands that interconnect the vertebrae to hold them in place. Ligaments are stretchable and flexible, to a certain extent. They come in various lengths and thickness. There are many, many ligaments in the neck and back running from one level to another. Some are very short, running only from one vertebra to the next. Some are quite long, extending the entire length of the vertebral column. Some are so small and thin you can almost see through them. The ligaments in the low back are the thickest because of their weight-bearing role.

Ligaments have an excellent nerve supply, meaning that if injured, torn, or irritated, they hurt. If stretched too far, they may break or tear.

When torn, the ligaments may heal; the ends may grow back together, with the formation of scar tissue. This scar tissue itself might be irritating to the sensitive nerves in the ligaments. Moving may hurt because it stretches the ligament and scar tissue. Unfortunately, the scar tissue that forms in or around the ligaments may not be as flexible and elastic as the original, uninjured ligament. It may never return to exactly as it was before the injury, but it needs gentle, consistent movement to become and remain as healthy as possible. If we don't move the ligaments, they get used to being held in one position or get used to less movement than they might be capable of. They hurt if moved beyond this, but the hurt may not be truly very "protective". Consequently, with this type of injury, gradual stretching and bending exercises are necessary to restore mobility to that part of the spine. This may or may not work completely, but usually needs to be tried as part of the treatment process.

Ligaments might be likened to a plastic drink can container. If given a sudden yank, they might snap, or simply be stretched too far. Ligament is not plastic but rather a living tissue that does heal. Usually it takes several days to weeks for injured ligaments to heal. However, pain can persist beyond that time because of scar tissue formation, inflexibility of the body part, and muscle spasm around the injured area. During this time continued exercise and mobility training are important to prevent spine inflexibility.

Muscles

The muscles are the body's motors. They move things, namely, body parts such as arms and legs. Using the physical principles of levers and pulleys, they move one bone in relation to another bone across a joint.

All regions of the spine are endowed with a bountiful amount of layered muscles extending from the neck down to the low back. The muscles work together across the vertebrae to provide smooth, powerful movements of the spine. Additionally, other large muscles like the trapezius are anchored along the spine to move the arms, head, and legs. Like ligaments, some muscles are very short, extending from one vertebra to the next; others are quite long, running almost the entire length of the spine. In addition, some muscles are not as deep and extend over the entire back, such as the trapezius muscle.

Muscles can hurt due to the prolonged extreme contraction which accompanies a spasm, like during a "charlie horse." Pain is produced because of reduced blood circulation during muscle contraction. Also metabolic by-products such as lactic acid build up during muscle spasm. These metabolic waste products irritate muscle fibers causing pain. The majority of back and neck pain is due to reflex muscle spasm. Direct muscle injury, or injury to the fascia (the membranes or bands or sheets of connective tissue surrounding bundles of muscle fibers) is also very common.

Nerves

The supporting structures of the spine listed above protect the two nerve elements found in the back and neck - the spinal cord and nerve roots. Outside of the supporting structures are the peripheral nerves. Injury to these parts may result not only in pain but also significant neurological problems such as weakness and numbness.

The spinal cord is the major trunk line between our central controlling station, the brain, and the body. All messages from the body sensed by the brain and all commands from the brain to the arms, legs and trunk pass through the spinal cord. This is why damage to the spinal cord results in loss of feeling (analgesia) and lack of movement (paralysis) to the body below the level of injury.

Because the spinal cord is so vital, it is well protected within the spine; it is located within the vertebral canal, the tunnel formed by stacking of the vertebrae. In addition, a series of coverings, called meninges, surround the brain and spinal cord. Three layers of meninges - dura mater, arachnoid, and pia mater - extend downward from the brain to envelope the spinal cord as it rests within the vertebral canal. The meninges are supplied by nerve fibers and - guess what - are painful. The condition of meningitis, an inflammation of the meninges due to an infection, causes severe pain.

The spinal cord is further protected by a liquid bath called cerebrospinal fluid. Cerebrospinal fluid is a clear, colorless, watery liquid that is actually made within chambers of the brain from the blood by a special filtration process. This fluid flows out of the brain within a subarachnoid space between the brain and meninges and down around the spinal cord. We make use of the cerebrospinal fluid and subarachnoid space to perform certain diagnostic tests such as spinal tap and myelogram. More about these later.

Like the vertebrae, the spinal cord is divided into numbered segments by regions - cervical (8, one more than the number of cervical bones), thoracic (12), lumbar (5), and sacral (4). Early in life, our spinal cord extends the entire length of the vertebral column such that the cervical, thoracic, lumbar and sacral levels of the spinal cord match those corresponding levels of the vertebral column. When we start to grow, however, the vertebral column grows much faster than the spinal cord. As a consequence, by the time

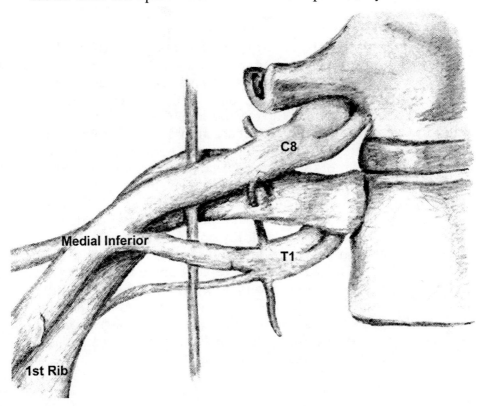

we reach adulthood, the spinal cord is much shorter than the vertebral column. The very end, or sacral level, of the spinal cord is about at the level of the L1 vertebra which is above the waist line. The meningeal sac containing cerebrospinal fluid, however, continues down the vertebral canal to the sacrum, containing only cerebrospinal fluid and nerve roots on their way into the legs.

Why is this point important? Well, for one thing, we know that injury to the low back will not result in damage to the spinal cord, simply because there is no spinal cord there to injure. Secondly, this construction allows us to perform certain tests such as spinal tap and myelogram without injuring the spinal cord for the same reason - no spinal cord to injure.

When a spinal tap is performed, a needle is placed between two vertebrae in the low back region, usually between the L3 and L4 spinous processes. The needle is gently advanced forward until the meningeal sac containing cerebrospinal fluid is reached and punctured. Depending upon the reason for the spinal tap, a relatively small amount of fluid, usually 5-10 cc, is drawn off, collected, and sent for laboratory analysis.

To put some perspective on this matter, the total volume of cerebrospinal fluid made in a day within the brain is about 500 cc, about one quart, or sixteen ounces. The total volume of fluid within the spinal fluid (subarachnoid) space around the brain and spinal cord is about 150 cc. In other words, we make over three times more spinal fluid each day than we have room to store. The excess fluid is reabsorbed back into the circulatory system in the head. This system results in a steady flow of spinal fluid from the brain, down around the spinal cord, and back up to the head. Since typically only 5-10 cc of spinal fluid are taken off with the spinal tap, you can readily see by these numbers that this fluid volume is rapidly and easily replaced. A myelogram is performed very much like a spinal tap, but instead of only taking fluid out, dye which is seen on x-ray is injected into the spinal fluid (subarachnoid) space. Myelograms are not being done as much as in years past because of other tests like CT and MRI scans.

At the other end of the spinal cord, the cervical region, the spinal cord joins the brain in a continuous flow of pathways and nerve tissue. The meningeal coverings also extend in a continuous fashion from the spinal cord up and around the brain. The junction of the spinal cord and brain occurs where the skull rests on top of the first cervical vertebra, called the atlas.

Nerve roots are the connecting link between the spinal cord and the body. The nerve roots are of two basic types: sensory and motor. The sensory nerve roots bring information into the spinal cord from the body. They provide sensory input to the brain via the spinal cord about our environment as detected by countless body sensors regarding touch, temperature, pain, and position sense (proprioception). In other words, everything that we feel is relayed by the sensory nerve roots. Motor nerve roots send information from the spinal cord out to the body, going primarily to muscles for body movements. Without proper functioning of the motor nerve roots, we would be unable to move our arms or legs resulting in paralysis. Polio is a condition in which the motor nerves to muscles are diseased, causing the muscles to stop working and deteriorate. Also, some motor nerve roots contain autonomic fibers (part of the nervous system that controls things automatically, things that we don't have to think about) which regulate blood vessels and sweat glands in the skin as well as visceral organs such as the heart, lungs, intestine, and bladder.

Nerve roots are connected to the spinal cord in a very organized fashion. Each spinal cord level has two paired nerve roots, one pair on each side - a sensory and a motor nerve root. The sensory roots, called dorsal nerve roots, are located toward the back part of the spinal cord while the motor nerve roots, called ventral nerve roots, are located toward the front part of the spinal cord.

Nerve roots are numbered by their associated spinal cord level. For example, the seventh segment in the cervical portion of the spinal cord is called C7. Consequently, the dorsal and ventral roots associated with this level are called the C7 nerve roots. Why is this important? A person with a herniated disc very often has the nearby nerve root affected by pressure of the disc on the root. For example, if you have a neck pain with a herniated C6-C7 disc (the disc between the sixth and seventh cervical vertebrae), the disc may press upon the C7 nerve roots causing pain, numbness and tingling down the arm (sensory damage) or weakness of the arm (motor damage).

The dorsal (back side) and ventral (front side) nerve roots join at each spinal level. In the cervical (neck) and lumbar (low back) regions, the individual nerve roots further join and intermingle in a very complex way to form a plexus. In other words, the nerves come out of the sides of the neck one at a time, but join in a bundle of nerves deep in the shoulder and chest to form the "brachial plexus" of nerves. From the low back the nerves form the "sacral plexus". From the plexus, peripheral nerves form which go into either the arm (from the cervical levels) or the leg (from the lumbar levels) to control the sensory, motor, and autonomic actions of that extremity. As a result of this intermingling, each peripheral nerve contains contributions from several nerve root levels. Think of this arrangement as a railroad switchyard where trains are rerouted and distributed from a central point to other destinations.

In the cervical or neck region, the nerve roots from the C4 down to the T1 spinal levels join and intermingle deep in the shoulder region close to the neck to form the brachial plexus. The major peripheral nerves formed from the brachial plexus controlling the arm are the radial, median and ulnar nerves. The radial nerve runs down the back of the arm and forearm to the back of the hand. The median nerve runs in front of the arm, forearm and into the thumb, index and middle fingers. The median nerve is the one irritated or injured in "carpal tunnel syndrome", which we will discuss briefly later. The ulnar nerve runs along the inside of the arm, forearm, hand and into the little and ring fingers. Because of the ulnar nerve's surface location at the elbow, it is prone to injury causing tingling into your hand when you hit your elbow (the "funny bone" effect).

In the lumbar or low back region, the nerve roots from the lumbar and sacral regions of the spinal cord (L1-L5 and S1-S3) join to form the lumbosacral plexus in the pelvic region. Two major nerves extending from the lumbosacral plexus to the leg are the femoral nerve and sciatic nerve. The femoral nerve generally runs to the front of the thigh, not going past the knee except for some sensation along the inside of the leg. The sciatic nerve runs down the back of the thigh. The term "sciatica" refers to the distribution of pain and tingling along this nerve. At the back of the knee, the sciatic nerve further divides into the peroneal and tibial nerves. The peroneal nerve runs down the front of the leg (shin) and top of the foot. The tibial nerve goes into the calf and sole of the foot.

Notes:

Chapter 2: ABNORMAL CONDITIONS

Types of Pain

Soft tissue injury, myofascial pain, musculoligamentous strain

Fibromyalgia

Fracture and dislocation

Mechanical

Nerve root compression

Degenerative conditions

Destructive lesions

Thoracic Outlet Syndrome

Carpal Tunnel Syndrome

Reflex Sympathetic Dystrophy

Temporomandibular Joint Dysfunction

Headaches

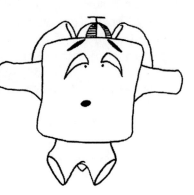

This chapter describes more things that cause the structures of the spine to hurt. There are many ways to discuss causes for neck and back pain. One way is to divide them into two major categories: spine and non-spine sources of pain. Spine pain can further be divided into traumatic and non-traumatic causes. First, a few words about various types of pain, including pain that is not always physical.

Types of Pain

A. Local: Pain can be very localized or focused in one area of the body. Examples might be a cut on the hand, a sliver, or a bruise on the hip from a fall on the ice.

B. Spasm: Muscle tightness around an injured area can be termed spasm pain. This can come on suddenly, gripping, knotting, and cramping. It can also come on more slowly. Often after car accidents or other traumatic events, a person may hurt worse as the hours progress. Sometimes by the next day the person can hardly get out of bed because of the tightness in their muscles.

C. Referred: Sometimes a specifically injured area of the body tends to send pain to another area of the body. This is called referred pain. A heart attack might refer pain to the left arm. There are no nerves that go from the heart to left arm, but still the person may feel pain in the arm from a problem in the heart. Irritating a particular nerve in the back of the head at the base of the skull (the greater occipital nerve) can cause pain behind the eye on the same side. The nerve does not go from the back of the head to behind the eye, but it can refer pain to this area.

D. Nerve root: Pain can travel along a particular path where a nerve goes. The nerve roots that come out from the spinal cord travel down the arm from the neck and down the leg from the low back. They travel very specific paths and distributions. Sometimes where you hurt can tell the doctor which nerve is involved.

E. Other: Pain is very complex and sometimes is not easily explained. How everything works in the body is not completely or perfectly understood. Not only are there many physical uncertainties, but also there are emotional and psychological factors that cause pain.

One might consider life stress pain, or difficulties dealing with losses or changes or uncertainties. One might consider pain associated with career difficulties. One might consider spiritual pain or existential issues like "Who am I, and why has this happened, and what should I do now?"

Also, is there "good pain" versus "bad pain"? Does just the right amount of exercise lead to "good pain?" But you don't want to do too much, too hard, too fast and cause "bad pain." "Bad pain" might signal tissue damage or at least the onset of a significant flare-up of pain. Does all pain really have a purpose? Is it always protective, and if not, is there some other purpose? These issues are discussed particularly in Chapter 4.

Most of the time, back and neck pain originates from the spine due to one or more of several problems caused by a trauma such as a falling or lifting injury, a motor vehicle accident, or other similar injury. The injury and associated pain is often superimposed on prior bad habits and poor lifestyle choices. These might include, but are not limited to, smoking, dubious nutritional choices, effortless exercise approaches, ineffective stress management techniques, and unsafe work habits, and not taking care of yourself. One patient said, "Always remember, your job is more important than you are."

The major types of traumatic problems resulting in spine pain are: *soft tissue injury, fracture, dislocation, nerve root compression, and mechanical pain.*

Soft tissue injury, myofascial pain, musculoligamentous strain

Soft tissue injury refers to damage to ligaments, tendons, and muscles in the spine. This sometimes might be called "musculoligamentous strain" or "myofascial pain". "Myo" refers to muscle and "fascial" refers to the connective tissue or bands of tissue that surround the bundles of muscle fibers. Most acute and chronic neck and back pain is due to injuries to these structures. For example, neck pain following a "whiplash" injury during a rear-end collision may be the result of soft tissue injury. Such an injury causes a localized irritation from tearing and stretching in ligaments, muscle fibers, and fascia. This irritation sets up a reflex muscle spasm, a response of muscle tightness surrounding the injured area and spreading outward from that area. The natural response of the body to such spasms is to guard and protect itself by holding that body part (i.e. neck) still. The resulting muscle contraction further aggravates the pain from the localized spasm, resulting in more spasm and pain. You can see that the proverbial vicious cycle developing, pain-spasm-pain-spasm-etc.

When an injury occurs in one place in the back or neck, the muscle around that area might become tight in order to protect the injured area, to allow it to heal, to hold it stiff and still, and to prevent further injury. When a muscle is held tight, it squeezes blood out of itself like water out of sponge. Hold your arm out straight at shoulder's height for a short while. You will notice that the muscle around the shoulder is being held tight in order to hold the weight of the arm up. The muscle begins to feel sore, telling your brain to let the arm go down in order to let more blood supply flow in and out of the muscle. You let the arm down and it feels better.

You can't hold the arm up forever. The muscle will become very tired because it needs more blood supply, oxygen, and glucose for energy. If it stays tight, it will become more and more tired as the arm feels more and more heavy and harder to hold up. Similarly, if your neck muscles are tight, your head might feel heavy.

If you try to run long distances when you are out of shape, your leg muscles will cram or tighten when they become tired. Tight muscles become sore and tired; tired muscles become tight; tight muscles become sore and tired; tired muscles become tight; and around and around it goes.

There may not be much reason for it to change. Heat, massage, ultrasound, and muscle relaxant medications give relief by relaxing the muscles, but it may be only temporary.

Sometimes the treatment provides long term or permanent relief, if it promotes significant healing. If, however, you only experience one or two hours of relief, the other twenty-two hours of your day may find your muscles tighter than they were before the injury.

Exercise, if done properly and most often in conjunction with passive conservative treatment approaches, can change this whole story. The muscles can become more relaxed long term. You may be able to do more activity without becoming so sore afterwards. This treatment approach may or may not work completely, but it has great potential to give long term benefit as well as temporary relief.

Sometimes myofascial pain syndrome is thought to be a confusing, unclear, "garbage can" diagnosis. But, in truth, it is a medical problem that is not well understood and is in need of further research. With few objective clinical findings, it is often associated with multiple pain complaints which may appear more psychological in origin. This disorder is suspect by some in the medical community and is a confusing topic to discuss. The confusion is legitimate because there are a number of inherent problems with this diagnosis, including what to call it. Is it myofascial pain syndrome, fibrositis, fibromyalgia, myofibrositis, myofascitis, musculoligamentous strain, soft tissue injury, tension myalgia syndrome, or myalgic rheumatism? Musculoligamentous strain or soft tissue injury are common terms used to diagnose the syndrome occurring after trauma. In more recent years the term myofascial pain syndrome is being used.

Along with a confusion of labels is a lack of objective clues identifying myofascial pain syndrome. There are no neurological deficits unless nerve entrapment is noted due to tightened muscles or other reasons. Patients with myofascial pain syndrome often have multiple psychological problems stemming from chronic pain and disability due to the injuries.

Myofascial pain syndrome has been described by Drs. Travell and Simons, in their two volume texts often used by physicians and physical therapists in understanding and treating these problems. These physicians documented specific objective clinical findings as well as specific treatment approaches that are effective in managing this disorder.

Myofascial pain syndrome is a disorder of muscle and connective tissue characterized by pain, muscle length shortening, referred pain, and autonomic phenomena. A key physical finding is the presence of trigger points. A trigger point is a hyperirritable (very sensitive) spot within a taut band of a skeletal muscle that is painful on compression and can give rise to characteristic referred pain, tenderness, and autonomic phenomena such as local temperature increases, sweating, and numbness. Myofascial trigger points are often thought of as localized areas in the muscle basically starving for oxygen. This localized energy crisis results in release of biochemicals which sensitize or irritate nearby nerves. These nerves then initiate motor, sensory, and autonomic responses. Muscles with trigger points are constantly in energy crisis.

Pain referral patterns are characteristic for each muscle. For example, a trigger point in the upper trapezius muscle (between your shoulder and neck) refers discomfort to the posterior lateral neck (back and to the side of your neck) and temple. A sternocleidomastoid (large muscle front side of your neck) trigger point refers pain to the occiput (back of your head), forehead, and facial areas. Scalene (triangular shaped muscles deep inside the neck) trigger points give rise to discomfort in the arm and medial scapular(mid upper back by the shoulder blade) border. Location of discomfort follows predictable referral patterns and assists in location of dysfunctional muscle groups and active trigger points.

Trigger points can be active (pain and tightness) or latent (tightness only.) Trigger points are localized areas where the muscle contracts so much that it may cause a knot that you can actually feel under the skin. These painful areas can persist for a long time - sometimes years - and are usually not easily treated by conventional forms of physical therapy. A trigger point is like having a "charlie horse" in that area of muscle that just doesn't go away. The trigger point serves as a source of pain, resulting in reflex muscle spasm by the surrounding muscle fibers with improper body activity. Typically, when the doctor is examining you, deep pressure in the region of a trigger point can cause such pain in that area that it causes you to wince - resulting in the "positive jump sign." Sometimes pain as well as a tingling sensation can extend down an arm or leg from the trigger point, a phenomenon called referred pain.

Muscle overload, strenuous activities, fatigue, muscle overwork, emotional distress, anxiety, and trauma resulting from recent or remote past injuries can cause muscle tightness and myofascial trigger points. Often, when maintaining one position for extended periods of time, or with repetitive overuse, muscle tightness becomes a major problem.

Symptoms of myofascial pain can be fairly rapid in onset, such as following injuries or muscle overload. Symptoms can be gradual in onset, such as following muscle fatigue or muscle tightness from a long stressful period of time. Pain is usually described as steady, deep, and aching. Burning sensations are common. Muscle stiffness may be worse in the morning or cause restless sleep. Strenuous activity or even activity which seems relatively easy may cause worsening pain. The weakening of muscles containing trigger points is also very common.

There are no standard medical tests to identify this problem. The diagnosis is made by history and physical examination. The fact that there are not any tests available to diagnose myofascial pain has led many physicians to disbelieve the existence of this problem.

In terms of treatment, the first task is to ascertain the diagnosis and to rule out other causes of pain, such as a herniated disc. After the diagnosis is made, contributing factors for myofascial pain are investigated. Treatment of trigger points is most successful when the contributing factors can be eliminated or modified.

Myofascial pain syndrome is a regional disorder. The discomfort of myofascial pain is noted in specific regions of the body such as head, cervical, shoulder, or low back areas. This is in contrast to the generalized discomfort of fibromyalgia which is often felt in widespread areas of the body.

Characteristically, pain from soft tissue injury is a constant, nagging sensation that is always there. It feels localized in the muscle, particularly in the back of the neck, along the shoulders at the base of the neck, down the back along the shoulder blades, or across the back. It may be on one or both sides. Any type of activity such as repetitive bending of the head or back, lifting, and even temperature change such as cold weather may increase this pain. It usually increases as our day's activities increase muscle use, and thus the amount of muscle spasm.

The diagnostic criteria for myofascial pain syndrome are listed below. To diagnose myofascial pain, there should be the presence of all five of the major criteria, and at least one of the other criteria.

The management of myofascial pain is two fold:

1) *Identification and management of perpetuating or contributing factors*
2) *Direct treatment of the injured muscle.*

Identification of perpetuating or contributing factors is very important. Perpetuating factors are predisposing conditions which contribute to the persistence of trigger point activity. Myofascial pain contributing factors include mechanical factors and nutritional factors. They include diseases that may cause a decrease in metabolic or endocrine function. They may include chronic infection that may increase trigger point irritability. Psychological factors may hinder trigger point treatment by keeping the muscles in greater tension than they should be.

Mechanical stresses include body asymmetries and poor postural habits. Poor postural habits place considerable stress on injured muscles. Simple aids such as lumbar supports, cervical pillows, and chairs with proper back, elbow, and leg support can be a significant benefit. Protraction of the head, or holding the head forward can result in neck muscle tightness. Loss of normal lumbar lordosis, or flattening of the normal curve of the low back may be another postural habit which needs to be unlearned and retrained. Holding the head and neck in forward flexion for extended periods of time, or holding the neck in extension, looking up too much, can also be a strain on the neck muscles and fascia, ligaments, tendons, and joints. Mechanical factors may include poorly fitting furniture at work or home, poor posture such as slouching too much, sustained or repetitious muscle contraction, excessively quick jerking movements, immobility with muscle in shortened position, dental mal-alignment or grinding of teeth (TMJ, temporomandibular joint), straps, purses, or bras pressing on trigger points. There may be other mechanical factors or problems, some of which may be important, and others that may not be so important. These include short arms in relationship to body torso, long second toe, pelvic tilt (one side of the pelvis being smaller than the other), leg length differences, and scoliosis.

Nutritional deficiencies include inadequate intake, malabsorption, and increased demand of essential nutrients. Nutritional factors include inadequate or poorly digested water soluble vitamin intake as well as increased demand for these nutrients. Water soluble vitamins and sources include B1 (thiamine) found in pork, beans, nuts, whole grain cereals, kidney, liver, beef, eggs, and fish. B6 (pyridoxine), another water soluble vitamin, is found in liver, kidney, chicken white meat, halibut, tuna, bananas, yeast, eggs, whole wheat, and milk. B12 (cobalamin) is in liver, kidney, shellfish, other fish (to a lesser degree), poultry, egg yolk, and fermented cheeses. Folic acid is found in leafy vegetables, yeast, liver, uncooked fruit, fruit juices, and lightly cooked fresh green vegetables. Vitamin C (ascorbic acid) is very important;excellent sources include raw broccoli, brussel sprouts, collards, kale and sweet peppers, cabbage, potatoes, and citrus fruits. Minerals and trace elements such as calcium, magnesium, potassium and iron are also important. Two to four servings daily from the milk group is good for the amount of calcium needed. Good sources of magnesium are lentils, dark green leafy vegetables, fish or shellfish, wheat germ, and whole wheat bread. Potassium is in fruits, potatoes, green leafy vegetables, beans, lentils, nuts, and prunes. Iron is in lean meats, organ meats, green leafy vegetables, peas, beans, whole grain cereals, egg yolk and shellfish. The elderly and pregnant or lactating women may be prone to vitamin deficiencies. People with certain cultural dietary customs, substance abuse (alcoholism), crash dieters, economically disadvantaged, emotionally depressed, and people with serious illnesses may be prone to vitamin deficiencies.

Metabolic disturbances which affect the nutritional needs of the muscle may also be important. There are certain diseases that may cause a decrease in metabolic or endocrine function. These include hypothyroidism, anemia, hypoglycemia, diabetes, and gout.Infection, either acute or chronic, can be important. Viruses, bacteria, and parasites can chronically infect or infest the body and cause increased trigger point irritability. Viruses are commonly associated with colds, cold sores, and the flu. Bacteria may be associated with tooth abscesses, blocked sinuses, and urinary tract infections. Parasites are less common in our culture, but include tapeworm, giardiasis, and amebiasis (usually resulting in bloating, diarrhea or bloody stools).

Allergies, such as allergic rhinitis (hay fever) that result in a runny nose, watery eyes, and sneezing, can aggravate myofascial pain syndrome.

Impaired sleep patterns are very common and can also have significant effects on myofascial pain. It is sometimes thought that if one did nothing else except help a person sleep better, there would be significant success in lessening myofascial pain. Myofascial pain, of course, can cause impaired sleep as well.

Emotional distress is much more significant than many people think. Psychological factors that will hinder trigger point treatment include poor understanding of the problem, depression, anxiety, worry, guilt, anger, blame, fear, and many other emotions that tend to make one feel "up-tight." Holding these emotions inside with little or no expression is not helpful in dealing with myofascial trigger points. Also denying that psychological factors play a part in precipitating or perpetuating myofascial pain will not help one to overcome or deal better with these problems.

Nerve root impingement by herniated disc, arthritis, or other causes of nerve entrapment or nerve irritation are factors that might cause or perpetuate trigger point discomfort. The underlying problem results in the response of muscle tightness to protect or hold the area still. This, as stated previously, results in more pain, and again in more tightness, a vicious cycle.

The second approach in dealing with myofascial pain is the direct treatment of the injured muscle. Myofascial pain is a disorder caused by trauma. Trauma can either be obvious and severe, sometimes called macro-trauma from a known injury, or it may be less obvious, sometimes called micro-trauma from repetitive overuse injuries or poor postural habits. Myofibrils, or small fibers in the muscles, are torn as a result of the injury causing a leakage of calcium into the muscle tissue. Calcium causes a strong contraction which if sustained, depletes the tissue of its main energy source. This energy source is called adenosinetriphosphate (ATP). At the microscopic level muscles are made of very tiny chemical filaments called actin and myosin. Imagine gradually folding your hands and fingers. When they are apart it is like the stretched out, elongated muscle. When the hands and fingers are folded together it is like the muscle that is contracted. The normal sliding mechanism of myosin and actin is dependent on ATP. Without this energy source the fibrils no longer slide efficiently and become locked upon each other creating a physiologic contracture. This might be similar to folding your hands and fingers tightly and holding them so they will not come apart. The contracted area is therefore energy deficient and becomes hypoxic (lacks oxygen). It does not allow for normal blood circulation to receive blood supply and energy and to get rid of its waste products like lactic acid and carbon dioxide. This results in taut bands and shortened muscles. The patient's mobility is severely affected.

To lessen the calcium leakage or lessen the underlying painful stimulus may be important. However, the key to treatment is mainly to restore normal muscle length by stretching and unlocking the myofilaments. Once that is accomplished, nutrients and oxygen can again bathe the injured area, restoring and replenishing the ATP energy reserves.

The patient should understand that stretching, at least initially, may be an uncomfortable process. Stretching can be greatly facilitated by the use of fluori-methane spray or similar approach. Fluori-methane spray is a fluorocarbon vapo coolant. The spray is directed over the length of the muscle and over its pain reference zone, or main are of pain. The cool spray is distracting. This inhibits the pain perception or experience that the person is used to. Since the pain is not appreciated as much when it is numbed somewhat by the cold, the muscle might be carefully and slowly stretched out more without the resulting response of muscle tightness or contraction.

Along with stretch and spray, ultrasound, acupressure, and myofascial release techniques are helpful adjuncts in stretching muscle fibers. It is imperative that you use a home stretching program. This will help you obtain mobility by postural education and regaining control of the pain problem. The length of the physical therapy varies from individual to individual. Generally, physical therapy is used 2-3 times per week for 3-4 weeks. Often therapy is extended for an additional 3-4 weeks with a gradually tapering schedule. During the last 1-2 weeks, you might be going only once a week. This serves as close follow-up to make sure you are retaining increased muscle mobility as well as not suffering any major setbacks. Stretching muscles containing trigger points must be performed frequently through the day in order to maintain optimal muscle length and prevent reactivation of trigger points.

Trigger point injections may also be quite useful and helpful in the treatment program. Trigger point injections are technique sensitive. In other words, the active trigger point and any satellite or surrounding lesions need to be injected in order for it to work properly. Often 1% Xylocaine is used because of its safety and availability. Procaine is more often noted in the literature, but it is not readily available. A small amount is used, approximately 0.5 to 1 cc of the 1% Xylocaine solution. The trigger point is injected and the needle is directed in a circular pattern around the trigger point. Xylocaine has a vasodilatory (dilating blood vessels) effect on the trigger point increasing capillary (very small blood vessels) circulation. It also has a curarae-like action on the myofilaments (very small fibers of muscle). This relaxes the taut band and releases the physiologic contracture within the muscle. Following the trigger point injection, the taut band may be more supple and trigger points may no longer refer pain to other areas of the body. Cortisone is usually not used in combination with the Xylocaine because there is little, if any, histological evidence of an inflammatory process within the trigger point. There is also the risk of systemic absorption (absorption through the whole body) and muscle necrosis (shrinking or dying of muscle fibers) with the cortisone. These problems typically do not occur but certainly could. Cortisone/xylocaine combination has been used in the past, but it may not give any additional benefit over the use of Xylocaine alone

The treatment approach is therefore directed at diagnosis, identification of perpetuating or contributing factors (including emotional responses and psychosocial stressors), a course of physical therapy, trigger point injections, and most importantly, a home stretching and exercise program. Prevention of trigger point reactivation is dependent upon addressing contributing factors and maintaining optimal muscle length.

Myofascial pain syndrome is a complex disorder which may need a comprehensive pain management approach. An exercise program is part of this approach. Once you regain mobility, you need a conditioning exercise program to strengthen and build endurance. Specific body part exercises for range of motion, stretching, flexibility, relaxation and strengthening are very important. These usually have to be done in a very slow and gentle manner, especially at first. General body endurance building is also very important. Mental imagery for muscle control, pain control, sleep and stress management and control can also be extremely beneficial. Success is more likely if various treatment approaches are accomplished in a gentle, consistent, and gradual manner.

The goals in treating a myofascial pain problem include lessening the underlying noxious painful stimulus if possible, returning muscles to their normal length and tone, recapturing a functional life, and reducing the negative emotional effects, perceptions, and responses. Reduction in dependence on medical and the health care system is desired by almost everyone. It then becomes very important to address other specific goals of patients, family members, doctors, employers, insurance carriers, and others appropriately involved.

In summary, myofascial pain syndrome is a complex and controversial medical entity. There is much confusion about the diagnosis and treatment because of lack of specific tests to identify the problem clearly. Myofascial pain should fit definite criteria and should not be confused with other muscle pain problems. A treatment approach of restoring normal muscle length is important. It is also important to identify and treat perpetuating or contributing factors. The ultimate goal is to help the injured person lessen the pain as much as possible and to regain control of the pain and its effect on their lives.

Fibromyalgia

Another term, fibromyalgia, is often used to describe a disorder with similar but different symptoms from myofascial pain syndrome. Fibromyalgia is probably more common than is documented and may not really be a single discrete condition. "Myo" refers to muscle, "fibro" refers to the fibers in the muscle, "algia" means pain.

No one is sure about the specific relationship to other medical conditions such as rheumatoid arthritis. However, fibromyalgia may be an initial manifestation of hypothyroidism. It may also be related to viral illnesses, hepatitis, mononucleosis, and a fairly common heart condition called mitral valve prolapse (MVP). Fibromyalgia is not routinely diagnosed and the average duration of symptoms at the time of diagnosis may be 5 years.

Treatment may include non-steroidal anti-inflammatory drugs, tricyclic antidepressants, muscle relaxants, physical therapy, relaxation techniques, stress management techniques, and exercise programs. All may work to relieve some of the symptoms such as local pain, stiffness, and sleep difficulties. Steroids do not really work for this condition.

Tender spots of fibromyalgia are most often found at the insertion of muscle into bone, whereas trigger points of myofascial pain can be felt in the bulk of the muscle. A key is that myofascial pain is a regional pain whereas fibromyalgia is widespread. Also myofascial pain often occurs after trauma, whereas fibromyalgia may not be precipitated by trauma. The criteria for fibromyalgia include the following:

Major clinical criteria:

1. Chronic, generalized aches, pains, or stiffness: axial, upper, lower, bilateral parts of body.
2. Multiple tender points at characteristic locations: at least 11 of the following 18 bilateral areas: Occiput, Lower cervical, Trapezius, Supraspinatus, Second rib, Lateral epicondyle, Gluteal, Greater trochanter, Knees.
3. Absence of other systemic condition to account for these symptoms.

Other clinical criteria:

1. Disturbed sleep (morning fatigue and stiffness)
2. Generalized fatigue and tiredness
3. Subjective swelling and numbness
4. Pain in neck and shoulders
5. Chronic headaches
6. Irritable bowel syndrome
7. Deconditioning

Fracture and Dislocation

A severe injury may cause fracture to the vertebrae or dislocation of the facet joints. Usually this type of injury results from a serious motor vehicle accident or a fall. A lifting injury at work or even a whiplash-type injury from a low velocity rear end collision will most likely not produce this type of problem, but can lead to similar problems. After severe injury, x-rays may be performed during an emergency room assessment to evaluate the possibility of these problems. Chronic pain problems sometimes may be caused by these ongoing conditions.

Other than the severe local pain it produces, a simple fracture of the vertebra in itself may not result in serious consequences. However, a vertebral fracture may result in bony fragments which could damage the nearby spinal cord or nerve root and require decompressive surgery. If the fracture produces such instability that one bone slides upon another, this needs to be known immediately to prevent damage to the spinal cord. A tragic result from a broken neck, such as occurs during a diving injury in shallow water, is transection or severe damage to the spinal cord at that level, potentially causing permanent paralysis.

The bones can be fractured in an injury, and this might be seen on an x-ray, but an unseen bone chip could be irritating a nerve near it. When bone is fractured, the body tries to lay down calcium in and around the fracture site to help heal the injured area. "Bone spurs" or "osteophytes" may form as part of the body's healing process. These actually can cause problems themselves, irritating nerves and ligaments near them.

Dislocation of the facet joints may cause pain as well as limit the movement of the spine at that level. In this situation, the facets of one vertebra ride up on the facets of the next, locking them in place much like the bumpers of two cars caught in a collision. This condition can be seen on routine x-rays of that part of the spine. Because severe muscle spasm from injury can cause significant impairment of mobility, x-rays are needed to rule out such dislocation.

A joint can become swollen when injured. If you try to catch a football or basketball on the end of your index finger, you might jam the joints and end up with a swollen knuckle joint. If injured badly enough or repeatedly, the joint can remain swollen or enlarged to a certain extent permanently.

Mechanical

Mechanical low back pain results from irritation to the movable joints in the low back area, such as the facets and sacroiliac joints. Mechanical pain can be present in the neck resulting from irritation of the joints there as well. This type of pain comes and goes. With rest there is little or no pain. With movement such as bending forward and back or side to side, the pain becomes prominent in the back or neck areas, usually near the middle of the spine. Neither pain nor other sensations, such as numbness or tingling, course very far down the legs or arms. Often joint problems in the back send symptoms down into the buttock or thighs but not below the knees. The symptoms are diffuse rather than specifically localized and do not follow particular nerve root patterns. Facet joint problems also may result in pain when extending the spine or bending backwards. The person may have difficulty lying prone or on their abdomen because of the back extension. The person may have difficulty bending over the sink to shave, brush their teeth, or wash dishes because the joints are being held in an uncomfortable position for too long. Bending forward to pick something up off the floor might be fairly easy, but getting back up from that position may be very difficult.

A congenital - i.e. there since birth - condition of the spine termed spondylolisthesis often doesn't cause any problems, besides the occasional back pain. But with an injury, the spondylolisthesis may serve as a significant source of mechanical low back pain. This condition is due to lack of fusion of certain parts of the vertebrae during embryonic development. There are varying degrees of severity, usually graded I (least severe) to III or 1V (most severe). With this lack of fusion is a certain degree of instability of the lumbar region which causes slippage of one vertebrae upon the next. The more severe the spondylolisthesis, the more unstable the low back is and the more pain that is generated

Nerve root compression

Certain conditions such as a herniated disc and/or degenerative bone changes can result in compression or pinching of the nearby nerve roots. In addition to back or neck pain, the hallmark of nerve root compressive difficulties is that it produces symptoms down the corresponding arm or leg in specific nerve pathways.

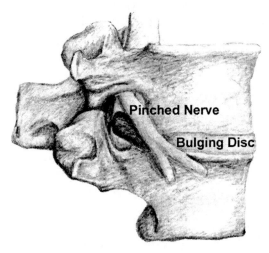

As we discussed earlier, each nerve root is distributed to specific regions of the body. A C7 nerve root, for example, runs down the back of the arm, top of the forearm and hand, and into the middle three fingers. Pinching of that root in the neck by a disc, therefore, causes symptoms of pain, numbness or tingling to shoot down the arm in that nerve root distribution. In addition, the C7 nerve root goes to specific muscle groups in the arm such as the triceps (pushes the arm out) and extensor carpi radialis (bends wrist upward). With sufficient injury to the nerve root, those muscle groups weaken because of poor nerve functioning.

Because of the potential for loss of sensation or lasting paralysis due to irreversible damage, nerve root compression is the most worrisome of traumatic spine conditions. Fortunately, most acute and chronic neck and back difficulties are not related to this problem.

Symptoms due to a herniated disc may develop immediately after an injury; the herniated disc placing direct pressure on the nerve root. Such symptoms may also develop later as the damaged annulous fibrosus gradually weakens. With time, a simple cough or twist of the body may be sufficient to complete the rupture, extruding the nucleus pulposus out of the disc. Quite characteristic with herniated discs, a cough, sneeze, or straining as with bowel movements increases the amount of radiating pain or other symptoms. These types of activities, termed Valsalva maneuvers, increase the pressure within the chest and abdominal cavity. This increased pressure causes more pressure on the herniated disc, resulting in increased pressure on the pinched nerve. The net results are increased symptoms of pain and numbness or tingling down the extremity in the specific nerve distribution.

Nerves themselves can be injured, stretched too far, torn, and bruised. They often take longer to heal than other tissues and structures in our bodies. They may take months or even as much as a couple years to heal depending upon what happened to the nerves. If a nerve is irritated or "rubbed on" by some other structure near the nerve, it tends to become swollen or "inflamed". There is only so much room for nerves in the first place, and if they become swollen they may get irritated worse and continue to be swollen, another "vicious cycle". Treatment is often directed at trying to decrease nerve swelling and irritation. Non-steroidal anti-inflammatory medications (Motrin, Indocin, Feldene, Naprosyn, Vioxx, Celebrex, Aspirin, etc.) can be used. Steroids (cortisones: Decadron, Prednisone) can be used by mouth or injection into a local area. Bed rest, traction, and physical therapy to relax muscles can all help decrease nerve irritation and swelling.

To recap, nerve root compression from a herniated

disc usually results in neck or back pain associated with pain, numbness or tingling in a specific distribution down the corresponding arm or leg. There may be weakness in specific muscle groups as well. Generally, these symptoms worsen with coughing, sneezing, or straining. Although the less common of traumatic causes for neck and back pain, this problem needs close medical and, if indicated, surgical attention.

Degenerative conditions (Aging)

Degenerative changes can occur after injury producing permanent changes in the bone structure. These changes are the body's response to local stresses from injury resulting in deposits of calcium anywhere along the vertebrae. These deposits are called spurs, producing a condition known as spondylolysis. If the spondylolysis is extensive enough to push on nerve roots, particularly at the intervertebral foramen, nerve root symptoms and/or damage can occur. Usually in these conditions, the original injury or a series of injuries occurred a year or so prior to the onset of symptoms. Sometimes no distinct neck or back pain is felt, but rather there may be nerve root symptoms such as numbness, tingling, or pain in the arm or leg. Muscle weakness may also result.

There are many diseases of the spine which produce back and neck pain, and may occur without any prior injury to the spine. These conditions can be serious, for they are often progressive and can lead to disabling problems. The purpose in writing this section is not to give a detailed description of these conditions, but rather to simply make you aware of them. The bottom line here is that significant spine pain without any obvious history of injury or trauma needs a thorough consideration of these diseases.

Arthritis is one of these conditions. There are many kinds of arthritis, but this book is simply describing the most common form that involves the spine. Arthritis means "inflammation in joints". "Arth" means joint. "Itis" means inflammation. Inflammation can occur in joints and cause a lot of trouble and pain. Osteoarthritis is a condition that involves the bones and joints in such a way that there may be extra bony growth around the edges of the bones and in the spaces between the bones, the joints. It is very common. All of us will get some of this as we get older. The discs tend to wear out and narrow causing the body to try and hold things still by making muscles tight and growing a little extra bone around the edges. It doesn't necessarily cause any symptoms but certainly can if the bony growth irritates any nerves nearby. Age, trauma, and wear and tear cause and aggravate this condition.

Ankylosing spondylitis is an uncommon condition involving the spine, joints, and ligaments surrounding the spine. In this, the ligaments harden or calcify to a certain extent. Men are affected more than women. Stiffness, limited motion, and a possible family history of early back pain are signs of this condition. Concurrent Reiter's syndrome (a condition with a specific triad of urethritis, conjunctivitis, and arthritis) could possibly be present. Psoriasis, inflammatory bowel disease, cauda equina syndrome (pinching or compression of many nerves down in the low back and tail area resulting in symptoms into the legs), sacroiliac joint degeneration, bony ridging of vertebral bodies (bamboo spine), vertebral bony destruction (late) may also be present.

Destructive Lesions

There are many types of cancers or tumors that can compress nerves or result in nerve involvement, pain, or other symptoms. These types of problems usually come on gradually and progressively. Many times tests and exams are done to rule out such problems. Tests may come back normal, which doesn't necessarily mean that there is nothing wrong or the problem is imaginary, but rather that it is probably true that things like this are not present.

Infections are also usually gradual in onset; tests and exams are also done to rule out these types of conditions.

Again if the tests are normal, it doesn't mean that nothing is wrong, but rather that this type of condition is probably not present.

Osteoporosis is the most common condition that we think about as a destructive condition. It involves a gradual reduction in bone mass and density. The matrix of bone minerals deteriorates gradually, especially as we get older, and in women much more than men. In the early phases there are usually no symptoms. But later on this can result in bone fractures, pain, and changes in body posture. Exercise, nutritional and calcium supplementation, and estrogen replacement when appropriate, are the main treatment approaches.

Thoracic Outlet Syndrome

Pain of the neck or back can originate from areas other than the spine. There are many conditions that might affect the shoulder, arm, or hand and result in pain in both those specific areas and also in surrounding areas. Pressure on nerves in the shoulder or arm can cause referred pain in the neck. A fairly common problem in this category as a consequence of injury is thoracic outlet syndrome. With this condition, pressure from muscle spasm around the neck, shoulder, cervical rib, extra rib at the top of the rib cage, fibrous bands of tissue, or even scar tissue after injury can irritate and injure the brachial plexus. In addition to neck pain, typical symptoms include numbness and tingling along the inside of the forearm and hand and into the ring and little fingers. Cold, burning, prickly pins and needles sensations and weakness can occur. Raising arms into the air as in combing or brushing the hair increases these symptoms.

People who sleep with their arms over their heads are at risk for development of symptoms, but house painters, hairdressers, and truck drivers also may develop problems because of the position of their arms above the shoulders. The condition may also occur due to muscle tightness around the area after neck or upper back trauma.

Treatment consists of conservative measures such as physical therapy and stretching exercises, or surgical removal of the first thoracic rib or congenital rib. Conservative measures are effective 70 percent of the time.

Carpal Tunnel Syndrome

Another example of nerve pressure which may cause neck pain is carpal tunnel syndrome. In this condition, the median nerve as it runs through the wrist may be compressed within the wrist. Typically carpal tunnel syndrome causes numbness, tingling, and pain into the thumb, index and middle fingers which awaken the person at night or occur while using the hands or driving. Weakness in the distribution of the median nerve can also occur. Pain in this situation can be referred into the arm, shoulder, or neck.

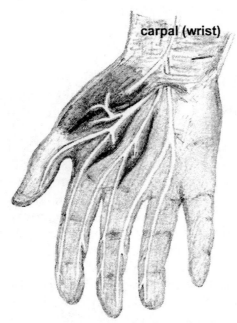
carpal (wrist)

There are actually three main nerves that go into the hand from the arm: radial (to the thumb), median (to part of the thumb, the index, third and part of the fourth fingers), and ulnar (to the fifth and part of the fourth digits). The median nerve goes through a tunnel of connective tissue in the middle of the front part of your wrist (carpal area). Sometimes the tunnel can become narrowed, for various reasons, and pinch or damage the median nerve. If the problem is present, it should be observed closely by your physician, watching for any progressive nerve damage. Clinical examination and EMG can help in this monitoring process. Discontinuing the excessive overuse, misuse, or trauma of the wrist and median nerve can be part of the treatment plan, and if needed, surgical intervention can be accomplished.

Reflex Sympathetic Dystrophy

Reflex sympathetic dystrophy is a short-circuiting of the part of the nervous system which is not normally under conscious control. This is the "autonomic nervous system" which takes care of things "automatically". The sympathetic nervous system, a part of the autonomic nervous system, is responsible for regulating bodily functions such as the temperature and circulation of our extremities, blood pressure, muscle tightness, sweating, and many other functions. The sympathetic nervous system is "in sympathy" with the environment (i.e., if you cut your hand, the blood vessels constrict to help stop the bleeding). Its role in the maintenance of blood flow to the skin and muscles of the limbs is where our interest is focused. Due to a major or minor trauma, the sympathetic network may become hyper-excited. If it does, the network responds with a reflex vasoconstriction of small blood vessels in the extremity. This response is not a problem unless the sympathetic receptors don't return to their normal state, allowing for passive vasodilation (dilating of the little blood vessels to let more blood into the area) and adequate blood perfusion or blood supply to the area.

The short-circuiting of the sympathetic nervous system or the continual hyper-excitement of the sympathetic receptors results in symptoms of pain, temperature changes (usually cold), sweating, abnormal hair and nail growth, and ultimately atrophy of the muscles and bones from disuse. Even though the limb may be cold, the pain may be described as burning or stabbing. The decreased blood flow results in decreased oxygen delivery to the area. The skin may be mottled. The temperature may be decreased. Waste products build up because of the lessened circulation. Fluid retention may occur in the limb. The person may be hypersensitive to touch in the area and exhibit avoidance behavior. There may be poor response to conventional TENS (transcutaneous electrical nerve stimulator); it may actually aggravate the pain.

This condition is estimated to be a problem in 10-20% of all people dealing with chronic long-term pain. This equates to 6-12 million people in this country. It is not a rare occurrence. The diagnosis is made by the physician at the time of the examination. The problem may be misdiagnosed since it can be a multi-symptom/multi-syndrome disease. Thermography may be the only diagnostic tool available to identify the temperature changes and document the pathologic involvement. A bone scan can be helpful also.

The most effective treatment for this disorder is medication to stabilize the circulation. Procardia or guanethidine are two drugs occasionally prescribed. Sympathetic nerve blocks can be helpful in the diagnosis and treatment of RSD. Sometimes surgery to cut the sympathetic nerve into the painful area is necessary. Treatment needs to focus on the return of the sympathetic receptors to normal tonic activity; in other words, they need to slow down. Normally electrical activity travels through little nerves to the blood vessels and results in normal vasomotor tone. This is the tone of the little muscles in the walls of the blood vessels. This controls the constriction and dilatation of the blood vessels. The electricity travels at a rate of about 1-8 pulses per second. If the pulses travel faster, at about 30 pulses per second, full activation (i.e. vasoconstriction) occurs. This is the problem. When the nerves are irritated, the electrical pulses are too fast.

A particular TENS unit, Spectrum Max-SD, stimulates sympathetic receptors with a pulse rate more like their own normal signal. This unique pulse aids in slowing hyperactive receptors and breaking reflex vasoconstriction to return to normal vasomotor tone.

Temporomandibular Joint Dysfunction (TMJ)

This is the joint or space between the temple of the head and the mandible or jaw bone of the face. This joint can be hurt just like any other joint. It is injured sometimes in "whiplash" accidents when the head is thrown about rapidly. It can become painful if the muscles around the neck, head, and face are tight after injury. The joint can become painful if one grinds their teeth too much. This often occurs the night after a person has been under extra stress during the day, or if the person is holding in long-term stressful feelings and having difficulty dealing with stressful issues. The jaw bone and TMJ can become mis-aligned sometimes. There can be clicking in the joint, difficulty with chewing, or talking, and muscles around the neck and head can become tight in order to hold things stiff and still resulting in headaches. There is a disc of fibrocartilage in the joint cavity which can wear out or be injured and result in even more problems. Various exercises for the mouth and jaw and face muscles, various muscle relaxation techniques, stress management techniques, oral splint or mouth piece, and medications can often be used to give some relief, promote healing, and prevent certain problems. Sometimes surgery has to be done to correct the problem.

Headaches

There are only three main things that cause headaches. These include muscles that get tight, blood vessels that dilate or expand, and "everything else."

Muscle tightness occurs because of stress or tension in one's life or other physical reasons like neck injury. These headaches should probably be called "muscle contraction" headaches rather than "tension" headaches. The headaches, by definition, are always due to muscles being tight, but not necessarily due to tension in the person's life. Most of the time people have tension in their lives but do not have headaches associated with it. 90% of headaches are due to muscle contraction. The headaches may feel like a tight band around the head, or a pressure sensation about the head and neck. There are many clues to tell your physician that muscle contraction headaches are the problem. The treatments will include anything to help relax muscles temporarily or long term.

Vascular headaches or headaches due to blood vessels that dilate are also very common. Everybody has heard of migraines. There are many kinds of migraines. There are other kinds of vascular headaches also. Throbbing pain,

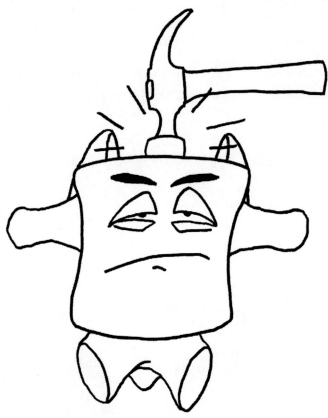

nausea, vomiting, sensitivity to light and sound, a strong family history, and many other characteristics might be clues to your doctor that vascular components to the headaches are involved. These headaches might be treated differently than muscle contraction headaches. Various medications can be used daily to help prevent them from coming on in the first place, or taken at the onset of the headache if there are significant warning symptoms, or taken to control the symptoms once they are full blown. Techniques other than medications, such as exercise programming, biofeedback, hypnosis, stress management, dietary alterations, and other changes in life style might have to be used.

The "everything else" headaches actually are rare occurrences but have to be ruled out. One has to make sure that there are no unusual problems such as brain tumors, or more common problems such as sinus infections, eye problems, dental problems, nutritional difficulties, drug reactions, etc. The physician can rule out these things and many more by means of the history, the examination, and if needed, ancillary tests.

Chapter 3: GENERAL IDEAS ABOUT PAIN

A lonely experience

Stimulus--Perception--Response

Endorphins

One's awareness and expectations with respect to pain can be helpful or a stumbling block when trying to get better. If you are not aware of the diagnosis and the realistic expectations with respect to treatment, you will not feel in control. This sense of confusion will contribute to your sense of separation from other people. Others will not understand.

Awareness that the painful stimulus is only part of the problem will be helpful. Gain knowledge. Lessen fear of the unknown. Learn how your own physical, emotional, biochemical, and behavioral responses are natural and understandable. Learn how they can be helpful or harmful. Learn what you can do to make a difference for yourself and for others.

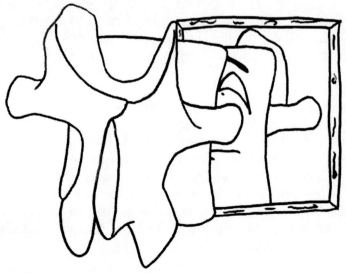

Pain is a lonely experience
(but not necessarily a private one)

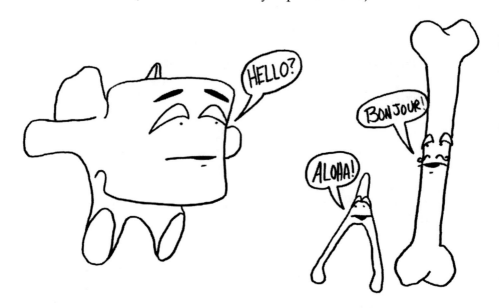

"Trying to express your pain to someone is like talking in a foreign language to them..." (patient's quote).

Pain is a very subjective, lonely experience. No one else feels pain the same as you do. Everyone feels pain differently. Your pain may fluctuate from hour to hour and day to day. You may have good days and bad days. Sometimes the pain bothers you more than it does at other times. In many ways, pain is very private. No one else can see inside you and really feel it, and it may be very difficult for you to express and describe to someone else what you are feeling.

One patient described it this way. "My family and co-workers had never suffered major back problems. In trying to share with them the pain, the frustration, I felt like I was standing alone in a desert where the wind blew away my words so no one could hear me, and the sand covered my footsteps, so no one knew I was there. But in this case, the people's apathy blew away my words, and their indifference covered my footsteps."

Most people do not develop chronic or long-term pain associated with an injury or other causes. Most pain problems are short term or temporary. This is what most people are used to. Therefore, society, in general, is very intolerant of long-term problems. People expect that the problems should go away in a relatively short time. If something lasts a long time, people tend to blame the victim. In psychology this is called "attribution error." People tend to attribute to the person, rather than the situation, the responsibility for their own difficulties. If, however, you are the injured person and you are feeling depressed, then you tend to also attribute to yourself the blame for your own problems. One might become more and more depressed, helpless, and hopeless. All of this is commonly seen in worker's compensation and personal injury systems. Employers, fellow employees, doctors, friends, relatives, and insurance companies frequently tend to blame the victim for their ongoing problems. Of course, they all may see themselves as victims for different reasons. No one really understands each other. The sense of being alone is ongoing but often unobserved and not understood.

Yet, sometimes the pain is not very private. Physicians, attorneys, employers, fellow employees, insurance companies, rehabilitation consultants, friends, and family members all invade your privacy in an attempt to understand what is going on and possibly help. They don't know what to do. You don't know what to tell them. All of this can be very frustrating. Awareness and communication eventually become very important factors in gaining a sense of control in these difficult situations.

Stimulus--Perception--Response (the painful experience)

To fully understand pain, we need to consider the important concepts of stimulus, perception, and response. The stimulus is what is wrong in your body. Perception is how this feels in your brain. Response is what happens to your body as a result of the perception of pain or what you do in response to having pain. All three of these things, stimulus, perception, and response, are important aspects of the painful experience.

Example: A person takes a needle, sneaks up behind you and sticks it into your buttock. The needle penetrating the skin is the stimulus. This message goes zinging up your spinal cord to your brain. When your brain receives the message, perception occurs. You raise your eyebrows and are definitely aware that something has happened that you do not like. This is perception. In response you might yell out--"Ouch!"-- and possibly jump up, clench your teeth and fists, and spin around to try to see what happened and try to prevent it from happening again. This is the "flight or fight" response. Your blood pressure goes up, your pupils dilate, you sweat, your pulse goes up, and your muscles tighten. You might run or hit the person who stuck you. This is all in response.

Let us change the example a little bit. The person takes the needle and waves it in front of your eyes but does not stick you. Your persecutor explains very carefully, dramatically, and sadis-

Stimulus

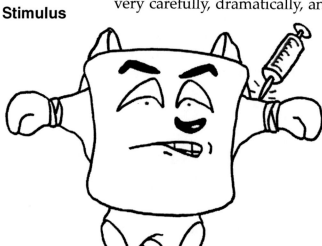

Fight

tically how bad this pain is going to feel. You may actually have the same response. Your blood pressure may go up, your pulse may go up, you may sweat, your pupils may dilate, your muscles may get tight, and you might make fists while shouting, "Oh, no you don't!" Yet, in this example there is no pain-producing stimulus. There is only the perception of possible pain resulting in the same type of response.

Which of the two experiences would you rather have? Would you rather be surprised or warned? Now you may prefer the first experience over the second or you may prefer the second experience over the first. You may prefer to be warned or you may prefer to be surprised. Everybody is different. But if you make a choice, this may tell you that the perception is important in how bad the pain experience really is.

When you go to the doctor, you want to find out what is the stimulus-- what is wrong in the body and what can be done to fix it. What can be done to make the stimulus go away? The physician's task is to discover the source of the stimulus (diagnosis) and to remove this source of pain (treatment). If the treatment does not fix the pain problem (stimulus), then you, the person experiencing pain, can diminish the intensity and severity of it by working on perception and response.

Let's examine these two concepts a little more. Perception is an individual picture of reality generated by

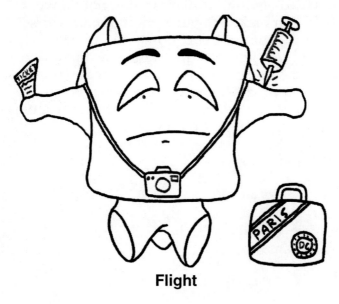

Flight

the brain. Perception involves different parts of the brain reacting to sensations. Many complex phenomena influence perception including judgment, early experience, emotions, anxiety, prior conditioning, attention, suggestion, and cultural background. If you are tired, rundown, lacking sleep, and/or experiencing a cold or flu, the perception of pain might bother you more. Pain might also bother you more if you are in a long-term, stressful situation. On the other hand, pain might bother you less if distracted by a different painful experience or other type of uncomfortable (or comfortable) feeling. A person may continue to have pain in a leg years after surgery to correct a herniated disc in the back. There may be scar tissue on the nerve or a small free fragment of disc, or disc space narrowing, or facet hypertrophy (overgrowth of small joints in the back or neck). The point is that even if pain has been present long term, it still can sometimes be worse or better. The basic "stimulus", underlying pathology in the back, may not really change much. The "perception" of pain can change frequently-- daily, sometimes hourly.

Fear worsens the perception of pain. If one does not really know exactly what is going on in the back, sometimes when the pain worsens, the person might be afraid something bad is happening. He or she may fear that the "stimulus" is worsening. It may or may not be worsening, but the "fear" can make the perception of pain worse. Fear might be good. It might encourage one to get it checked out. Pain might be good for the same reason. If one has it evaluated by the doctor, the problem might be fixable or at least the person might know more about what should not be done to make things worse. The fear of the unknown can make the perception of pain worse.

Patient's example: "*I was told I had a ruptured disc, but I didn't know exactly what that was. I only knew it hurt when I moved, so for months I practically stopped moving (as can be proven by the permanent couch button indents on my back!) With lack of movement, I gained weight, so I started walking. Then I heard that the ruptured disc could break off and press against nerves and kill me. So I stopped walking, I stopped moving, I almost stopped living. It's kind of a paradox, for fear of dying I stopped living. Thank God, someone recommended a pain specialist. I soon discovered that no, I could not die, and lying around was the worst thing I could do. Exercising and strengthening my muscles around the injury relieved some of the pressure and pain. If I'd only known the true facts, all those months of hell would not have been. Had I known the facts, I would not have fallen victim to misinformation.*"

Another thing that worsens the perception of pain is stress. It's not as though one opens up the paycheck and notices that it's $200 less than normal and instantly has a worsening of back pain. But if one has a lot of stresses going on in life, he or she might be more vulnerable. Pain may bother one more when under more stress. The effects of stress are so much greater than we recognize. Stress can be good and some people tend to thrive on stress. When pain happens, we may not be able to handle stress in the best way. With long-term pain we may not be able to do the things we used to do in order to vent stresses. We cannot do physically demanding, enjoyable activities. We then have more stress on board and fewer ways to vent, get rid of, or manage stress before the onset of pain. The feelings associated with pain may be stressful: anger, depression, frustration, guilt, worry, etc. Since pain is a stress, stress management techniques can be used to deal with pain, to lessen and better cope with the pain that remains.

How does the Guru lie down on a mat of nails or walk across hot coals? It is not because the nails are rubber or there are calluses all over his back or that the coals aren't really hot. He can do these things because he does something with his mind as well as his body to gain a certain control over perception and response. He blocks out pain or focuses on other things. He spreads his weight evenly or with balance.

A woman giving birth might practice breathing and muscle relaxation techniques to get through labor more easily. She learns with practice to focus on one thing at a time, to relax, and to make the pain more tolerable.

The mind is very powerful. One cannot "block out pain" if the pain has a purpose such as telling the person to check it and find out what is wrong. Nor can one block it out if the pain is protective, such as telling the person to take his finger out of a burning candle flame. However, if the person already knows what is wrong and has had it fixed as much as possible, blocking it out might be just the thing to do and might be very powerful and successful.

Think of the football player who sprains his ankle when he is on the winning team versus the one who sprains his ankle when he is on the losing team. Who hurts worse? The winner or the loser?

Imagine a 500 pound Bengal tiger coming into your room right now. Do you think you will get up slowly from your chair? No! Your brain will do what it has to do in order to survive. You will get up fast, and run fast in spite of pain. The anatomy (stimulus) stays the same. But perception changes.

A lot of things happen in response to pain. Many happen automatically. We don't have to think about them. A part of the nervous system called the autonomic nervous system controls the responses automatically. The autonomic nervous system is made of two parts, the sympathetic and the parasympathetic. These two parts work counter to each other. Sympathetic nervous system activation is what happens when an acute pain or stress is experienced. Imagine you are being stuck with a needle. Sympathetic nervous system activation can result in the following: *next page...*

1. *Fear, rage, fight, flight, alertness, vigilance (it would be hard to fall asleep)*
2. *Muscle tightness, muscle tension*
3. *Decreased blood flow, blood vessel constriction, to the internal organs and the skin and extremities*
4. *Sweating*
5. *Pupils dilate*
6. *Increased pulse rate*
7. *Increased blood pressure*
8. *Increased blood sugar*
9. *Increased secretion of epinephrine, adrenaline, into the blood stream*
10. *Decreased gastric acid production and secretion, but build up due to decreased gastric motility or activity*

With these responses, people can have a worsening of certain medical problems such as high blood pressure, diabetes or ulcers. When we are under stress (and pain is a stress), we can have more problems with these "target organs" as well as other body parts that might be weak or more vulnerable to the stresses in our lives.

Fear can cause actual symptoms. One patient was told to watch for bleeding from the kidneys. She was so fearful of this happening that within two weeks she was bleeding from the kidneys. Several extensive tests showed no probable cause for the bleeding. She was then told by another doctor that she was misinformed. Bleeding kidneys could not possibly be one of the symptoms of her disc problem. Within two days the bleeding stopped. Again, the mind is very powerful. It can work for us or against us.

One important response to pain is muscle tightness. Muscle tightness hurts. If we can figure out ways to control muscle tightness, we can control pain to a degree. We think of muscle tightness as our own body's protective response to something that is wrong. Initially, after an injury, the body attempts to hold everything stiff and still by muscle tightness, to protect it, let it heal, and prevent further injury. Muscles try to act like a cast on a broken leg. This is good at first, but after healing is done, it is no longer necessary. Yet muscle tightness may continue, and tight muscles continue to hurt.

Think of a sponge saturated with water. Muscle is saturated with blood. If we squeeze it tight, it is like squeezing the water out of the sponge. If one holds it that way too long, the muscle starts to hurt. This might only be a minute or two. How long can you hold your biceps muscle tight? Pretty soon it starts to hurt! The muscle begins to scream for a fresh blood supply and circulation to get new oxygen, sugar, and energy and to get rid of its waste products such as carbon dioxide and lactic acid. All we have to do is let the muscle loose for a moment and the blood circulates back through it, and it feels better again.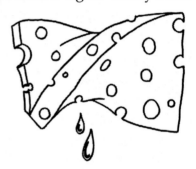

We can work and pump our muscles all day (once they get into basic shape). This tight-relax-tight-relax is all a muscle needs to have good circulation of blood and to keep working. Continued muscle tightness is more like the body's "overreaction." It causes more problems than it is worth. It hurts!

Think of an allergy. If pollen gets into the nose, most people simply sneeze. However, some people have allergies. Their bodies make all kinds of mucous and fluid and sends it into the nose and sinuses to wash out the pollen. The person holds his face in his hands and shakes his head slowly saying, "Stop with the mucous; I can live with the pollen."

With muscle spasm and tightness we might say the same thing. "Stop with the muscle tightness; I can live with a little irritation, scar tissue, bulging disc or whatever, but this muscle tightness is driving me crazy!"

Inflammation is part of a body's response to associated nerve irritation and/or muscle tightness. When one sprains an ankle, there are three things to do to lessen inflammation: *1. ice, 2. pressure (ace bandage - or the like), 3. elevation.* These steps are designed to lessen the influx of fluid and swelling. Swelling is one of the body's "overreactions" to the tissue irritation and injury. Often this response causes more trouble that it is worth.

If a muscle is held too tight for too long, portions of the muscle may be injured due to lack of blood supply. This area may heal and form a small lump of scar tissue, termed "fibrocytic nodule". This nodule can be painfully irritating and the muscle around it can be tight. Inflammation may occur, but typically is not present in these trigger points. "Trigger point injections" of novacaine-like substances and/or cortisone might help. The lump may remain. Usually it can't be cut out because scar tissue will probably grow back. Heat, massage, ultrasound, manual, myofascial physical therapy techniques, and other forms of conservative treatment may help relax the muscle around the nodule. Exercise and other stress management techniques can help strengthen, stretch, and relax muscles and prevent the muscle from getting tight so easily at times. When muscles get tight and stay that way for a length of time, they get tired. When muscles get too tired, they tend to tighten more and cramp. If one runs long distance when out of shape, leg muscles may cramp. the tired muscles become tight. If one holds an arm outstretched to the side, the tight muscles become tired. There is a vicious circle: tight muscles, protecting the injury, become tired and sore. Tired muscles become tight. Muscles are "smart," or almost seem to have a mind of their own. One might ask and try to make them relax, but they refuse to do so. They tell us to build strength and endurance gradually, consistently.

In addition to the many automatic responses, there are also behavioral responses such as saying "ouch", screaming, crying, yelling, swearing, grimacing, etc. One may do a lot of things, or act out our own responses.

Endorphins

A good response to pain is the production of endorphins. Endorphins are your own body's pain killing chemicals. They are made in certain areas of your brain. They are very good and very powerful. Endorphins are about 20-100 times stronger than morphine. Endorphins were discovered in 1969, and more and more is being learned about them all the time. When dealing with long-term pain, one needs to figure out ways to increase the amount and effectiveness of endorphins. One does not want to do things that tend to decrease nature's own pain killers.

Acute pain and stress increase endorphins. Long term pain and stress tend to decrease the amount or effectiveness of endorphins. If you hit your thumb with a hammer the pain is sharp, strong, and severe. The brain perceives the pain and says, "Holy mackerel, I better start making pain killing chemicals to help this person out! He is really hurting!" The brain quickly increases endorphins. Within a minute or so, the pain lessens somewhat and becomes dull, throbbing, aching, and less severe. This is endorphins at work!

If you were to go around all day hitting your thumb with a hammer, the pain in your neck or back might be less noticeable, but this, of course, is not the solution. You'll have lower levels of endorphins in the long run due to long-term thumb pain. Beginning slow, gentle, gradual exercises for your neck or back could be the answer even though it might hurt. You must understand your diagnosis and know in your mind as much as possible that you are not causing any damage. If you can know this and feel safe with the exercise activity, then you can go ahead and do the exercises for range of motion, stretching, flexibility, relaxation, strengthening, and endurance building. The key to safe exercise activity is to go very slowly, gently, gradually, and consistently.

Endorphins are also increased in endurance building. Long distance runners and swimmers might have more endorphins in their systems when they are in shape as opposed to when they are out of shape. Long distance runners get a "runner's high", thought to be due to endorphins. When one has pain he usually has less activity, decreasing endurance and causing endorphin levels to decrease.

Endorphins are thought to be decreased in someone with long-term pain and with long term stress. Think of it as though the brain tires of making and using them after a while. Endorphins are also decreased in amounts when we consume other chemicals like painkillers, some muscle relaxants, alcohol, excess salt, sugar, nicotine, and caffeine. These are stress producing chemicals. When we take a pain killer by mouth, our brain says, "Oh, I don't have to make these anymore." Unfortunately, the pain killers wear off after a short while and the perception of pain is actually worsened. The anatomy is the same, but the brain's and spinal cord's chemistry may be different. Compared to anything one can take in terms of chemicals from outside the body, the endorphins are much stronger and last longer in their effects.

Now that we understand the factors that influence the perception of pain as well as our responses, let's consider the different types of pain in the next chapter.

Notes:

_____

_____

_____

_____

_____

_____

_____

_____

_____

_____

_____

_____

_____

_____

_____

_____

Chapter 4: TYPES OF PAIN

Simple vs. Complicated

Acute vs. Chronic

Healing and time

This chapter addresses some very important ideas concerning chronic or long-term pain. Most people think of pain in fairly simple terms, "Find the problem, fix it, and be done with it." However many pain problems are not simple, are not of short duration, and will not go away by simply giving it more time. Many pain problems are very complicated in terms of clarifying the diagnosis, treatment options, and expectations for the future. Many pain problems last long-term, way beyond the healing phases, and may even last a life time. However, there is always hope. There are usually many things that can be done to change the situation and bring about improvements. Also, technology is always changing. Understanding the biochemistry, anatomy, and physiology of pain is improving.

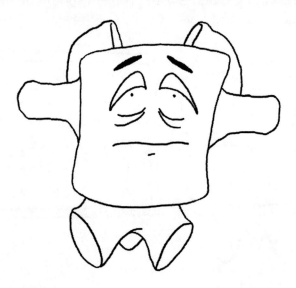

Simple vs. Complicated

Most pain can be classified as simple or complicated; acute or chronic. Simple pain is easily understood. This might be when you sit on a tack or hit your thumb with a hammer. It simply hurts and it does not need much explanation. You understand exactly what is going on and you do not want it to happen again. Simple pain is like getting a small cut and needing stitches. It may hurt for several days. In a week or so the stitches are taken out and that is the end of it, more or less.

Complicated pain is a different story. This type of pain may be difficult to diagnose clearly and is lacking in explanation. Not only is it difficult for the physician to accurately diagnose and explain, it is difficult for you to understand exactly what is going on. Complicated pain can last a long time. It can last beyond the normal time that it takes for healing. This pain is not only difficult to understand but it is also difficult to treat. The pain can also complicate your life a great deal. It can affect your activity, work, play, feelings, emotions, relationships, and behaviors.

This concept is important because often people come to the doctor expecting that the pain problem should be relatively simple to figure out and treat. Yet the diagnosis, treatment, and

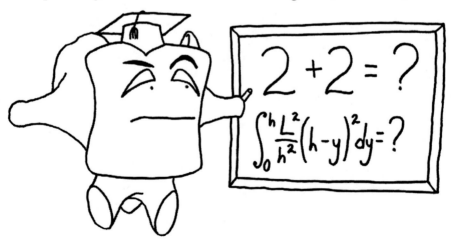

effects on the person's life may be very complicated. The frustration of expecting a simple answer or cure only makes the situation worse. It can be helpful sometimes to approach pain problems with the understanding and expectation that it could be complicated, requiring complex solutions.

Acute vs. Chronic

Acute pain is usually maximal at onset and relatively short-lived. Acute pain has a purpose--it is protective. It tells you not to do whatever it is that is causing the pain. It tells you to get your finger out of the candle or not to hurt your thumb with the hammer anymore (ie. when you miss the nail). Acute pain might be a sign that something is still healing. Healing after an injury may take time, usually fairly short: 6-8 days for a cut in the skin, 6-8 weeks for a fractured bone or a badly sprained limb. Some problems may take longer to heal: 6-12 months for injured nerve tissue; 1 -2 years for a brain injury. But all in all, most back and neck injuries heal in a few days to a few weeks. Pain may persist for months or years, but it may not be a matter of waiting around for things to heal. People often equate continuing pain with the need for continuing healing. However, many times the two are not the same.

In the acute phase it is usually true that things do heal better if given relative rest. Usually we don't keep walking around on a badly sprained ankle. We rest it to let it heal. The same is true for most fractures. We put a cast on it and walk around with crutches, giving the limb a rest and letting it heal. This takes a relatively short time, 6-8 weeks.

But back and neck problems often don't get the rest in the beginning that they might really need. We have to keep moving around to go to the bathroom, the refrigerator, and other important places. The neck is always holding up the head, which weighs 10-14 pounds, equivalent to a bowling ball. Muscles and soft tissue in the neck never quite get a good rest. The neck drags the head across the pillow at night. The back holds up the top half of our body. A broken bone usually needs rest at first. This is the usual for a simple fractured bone that needs immobilization for a short length of time. How long will it take to heal if we don't put a cast on it? It will take about the same length of time. It may take a little longer. It will heal. It may heal "crooked", but it will heal. This might be true of certain back and neck problems. They heal, but maybe when the healing is all done, they are not exactly the same as they were before the injury. They may be "crooked" or have scar tissue in sensitive places irritating nerves or causing continued muscle tightness, inflammation, ligament inflexibility, decreased mobility, and a decreased range of motion. These long term problems may lead to chronic pain.

Chronic pain is different than acute pain. Chronic usually refers to pain that lasts longer than 6 months. We might use the term to describe pain that lasts longer than the healing phase. Chronic pain does not have the same protective purpose as acute pain. It becomes more or less worthless. The pain in your leg years after surgery, due to scar tissue that cannot be removed from the nerve, is relatively worthless. It may be there all the time whether you cough, sneeze, run, jump, stay in bed, or whatever. It is not protective in general. It is just there.

Sometimes this same pain may change or worsen with certain activities. This may indeed be protective. This could be telling you not to do that certain activity, but the message can be a very difficult thing to discern. You may lift an object that is too heavy and the pain that you feel says to you "This is not a good idea." And so you put the object down. You have to listen to acute pain. You may have experienced pain that flares-up for seemingly no particular reason. You didn't lift anything wrong; you didn't sleep in the wrong position; you didn't sit too long in one place; there isn't any change in the weather; and you're not under any particularly different stress.   Therefore the pain becomes unreliable and relatively worthless.

The concept of good pain versus bad pain might be helpful here as well. Good pain might be that which you feel when you are using muscles, ligaments, joints, etc. to gradually get into shape. This might apply when you have not been hurt, or it might apply when you are doing activities even after being hurt, but you know the activities are safe physically. Bad pain might refer to what you feel when you are doing an activity that is not safe. It might refer to the pain you feel when you are unsure whether or not the activity you are doing is safe. Until you know the activity is safe, the pain might be considered bad.

Another patient used the term "working pain" versus "disability pain." The former refers to pain that is tolerable such that he could function. The latter refers to pain that is so disruptive that he could not function at all. This interesting concept points to the idea that the severity of pain may be dependent on many things. One might be the person's understanding or lack of understanding and fear of damaging something.

This is where understanding what is going on in the back or neck during those particular movements or activities can help you know if you are causing any damage. It can help to know if the activity is really worsening something or simply a continuation of the routine, long term, worthless pain. This is still very difficult to know many times, and sometimes simply cannot be answered completely. But if you go about your activities slowly, gently, gradually and "safely", you can gradually increase your activity level without causing the flare-ups of pain that lay you up for days or weeks and may even be a sign of tissue damage.

Chronic pain, long term, worthless pain, is indefinite in duration. One cannot tell how long it is going to last. It may last many months, many years, or a lifetime. It just keeps on going indefinitely, changing some with activities, the weather, stresses, and sometimes for no reason at all that you can identify. Some pain problems may lessen over many years. Long-term pain requires endurance building, while acute flare-ups might require relative rest. Endurance building is needed to do more activities with less pain. Relative rest can help in the healing phase, but once healing is done, then endurance building is necessary.

Healing and Time

How long does it really take? If a patient went to the doctor and asked about the continued leg pain ever since low back surgery twenty years previously, and if the doctor said, "These things just take time"...... This is the wrong answer. They might not know what the right answer is, but time might not have anything to do with it.

A patient might be told, "These things take three to five years." A patient might be told, "You'll be better in five to ten years." Sometimes these types of answers are correct. Sometimes the doctor might really have no idea what is going to happen over time. Often doctors don't like to say what is going to be "permanent" until at least a year has gone by since the injury. Or they don't like to say what is permanent until the appropriate treatment approaches have been tried. This might be true of soft tissue injuries, muscle-ligament strain, whiplash, and myofascial pain. Broken bones usually heal much faster than this one year time period. Brain or nerve tissue might take longer depending on the actual injury.

Since chronic pain is such a frustrating experience for the patient, family, doctor, and all concerned, let's examine this problem in greater detail in the next chapter.

Chapter 5: CHRONIC PAIN

Psychophysiologic Profile of the Person Dealing with Pain

Chronic Pain Syndrome

Results of Chronic Pain Syndrome: Changes That Occur

This chapter describes in a simplified manner a very complex pattern that might develop as a person is struggling with long-term pain. It is a typical pattern, but may not apply fully to you or your situation. It describes what is fairly natural and understandable. It also describes components of what people might call the "grief process" or very common experiences in dealing with loss. It discusses the development of numerous disruptions in one's life as the result of pain, yet also opens the door to various treatment approaches to bring about successful improvements and changes in these life situations.

Psychophysiologic Profile of the Person Dealing with Pain

A useful way to examine chronic pain is to see how it influences one's daily life. The following profile represents "normal" people and situations. This is you and me before pain comes on board. The pattern varies from person to person, since everyone is different, but basically our reactions and responses to pain are very similar.

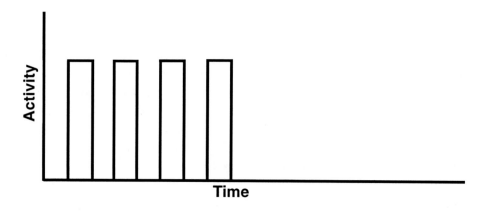

This bar graph represents 4 work days in your life before chronic pain. You start out early in the morning and work until evening. The work schedule may be different for each person. In general, this is an attempt to represent a certain "level of activity - work activity" for you before pain comes on board.

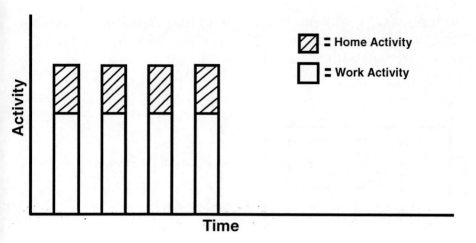

This graph (the stacked boxes) represents your level of activity at work and outside of work on each of the four days. This activity would include evening recreation. It might even represent work at home, like doing laundry, taking care of children, cutting the grass. This activity in combination with your work activity adds up to your total level of normal daily activity.

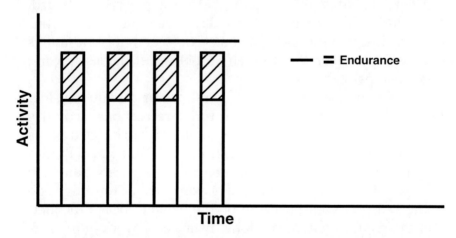

Your activity level holds up your level of endurance (the thicker, black line), stamina, or ability to keep going. Your endurance may reflect, to a degree, your ability to cope, both physically and emotionally, with life's irritations, problems, and frustrations. It is high when you are active, but not overwhelmed, with too much to do.

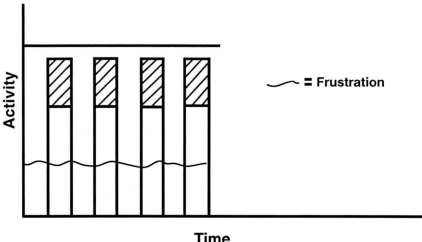

Time

This next line (the up and down, thinner line) represents your level of frustration with these irritations and problems of normal everyday life, again, before pain is on board. Frustrations fluctuate from day to day depending on numerous factors, different for each person. These may include things such as the weather, the children's problems, struggles at work, relationships, money, and so on.

You might keep your frustrations at a relatively low level by "venting" them with your fun or recreational activities much of the time. You may also talk them out; but activity is often a good way to manage frustrations. Your fun activities help in this way, but your work may also help, especially if it is physical work and/or you enjoy your work. You might go home and play your heart out on the piano or beat a racquetball against the wall, or run long distance, or work in the garden, or go dancing, or sew, or read, or many other things; and then you might feel better about your life and stresses to a degree.

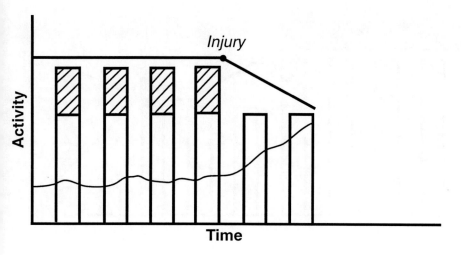

But when you're injured, things change. You may not be able to do the things you want to do physically because of the pain problem. You lessen your normal activity by cutting out certain things that hurt. Endurance begins to come down. Frustration begins to go up.

You may have to keep working because you need the income, but after work you don't go bowling when you are hurting like crazy. After work you may go home and rest. Again, everybody is different, and you may not be resting all that much. But you may have to cut out some activities, cut down on your normal level of activity, do things differently with less movement and enthusiasm. Consequently, your endurance level may drop as well.

Your frustration level goes up because you have fewer ways to vent your frustrations and stress, and you have more frustration and stress on board. Pain is a stress, and very frustrating.

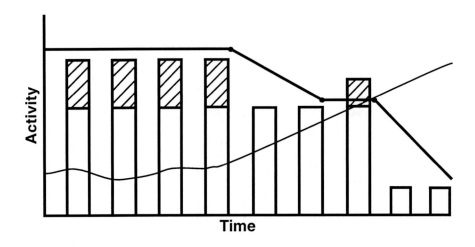

Time

Then somewhere down the line you try something that seems to be beyond endurance. You cut the grass, or do a little work in the garden, or shovel the sidewalk on a winter day. You try bowling one evening. Maybe you haven't done anything for fun for 2 or 3 weeks and your bowling team captain calls up and says, "C'mon, can't you go bowling with us tonight? We need you!" And you (grumbling to yourself, angry-frustrated, and afraid of the pain) say "Oh, all right, I will!" You say to yourself, "I'm hurting anyway. This resting hasn't really helped much. I might as well try it!" And so you go, but can only bowl one game. You hurt too much. You only get a 30 and cannot bowl the other two games. Your team has to forfeit and they don't want you back again -- or you're too embarrassed to go again. At any rate, very shortly, you pay for it with worse pain.

It may not require activity like bowling. It may only require simple or minimal activities like trying vacuum a room in your house. It might be as unassuming as writing a letter with your head and neck in forward flexion too long. It might be trying to scrape the ice off your windshield on a winter morning. It might be slow dancing at your cousin's wedding.

You end up with more pain after doing something

beyond endurance, and you may not be able to handle going to work. You may be hurting so much from this simple activity that you go to the doctor the next day and skip work. The doctor advises medications, physical therapy, rest, staying off work, or even going to the hospital. All this helps with the flare-up episode but not with the original problem.

After resting you feel somewhat better, less muscle spasm and slightly less pain, but also endurance comes down. If your only activity while at bed rest at home is going to the bathroom, raiding the refrigerator, and punching remote control on the TV, your endurance is going to come down.

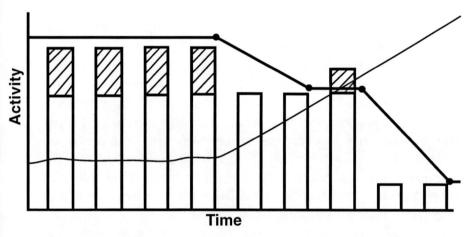

Then as you try to do activities, and the pain persists, frustrations go up. You are not sure what is really causing the pain. You don't know what to expect for the future. The more normal you try to be in your activities, the more you hurt. Treatment is only giving you temporary relief. You do feel somewhat better (with respect to the acute flare-up only) after resting for one or two days, or weeks, or months. You go back to the doctor and are advised to try going back to work.

The doctor may see that your frustration is way up, but then again you may be good at covering it up, and the doctor may not notice. You may wonder about his advice to go back to work. You wonder about no further diagnostic evaluation. You still do not really understand what is going on in your body. You are concerned that there are no further plans to treat or fix the problem. You wonder if the doctor thinks this problem is all in your head. As a result, frustration continues to stay high or even worsen.

You go back to work but it is beyond your endurance. The pain worsens and you can only handle half or three quarters or only a couple hours of work activities. You hurt too much. You go home.

Now things are really bad: no work, low endurance, high frustration, nothing for fun, no light at the end of the tunnel, and you may still not know really what is wrong with you in the first place. You feel miserable, afraid, angry, confused, and horribly out of control.

The hope is to reverse this whole process. To build up endurance in a very slow, gentle, and gradual way. If you go at the exercise plan too fast or too much, you most likely will only experience more pain and not really be able to build and improve. If you don't do anything, nothing will happen to change the situation. Therefore, to push beyond endurance just a little bit at a time, one day at a time, will most likely be successful.

Also, you will need to work on decreasing yourlevels of frustration. Gaining some success with the physical end of the issues will be helpful. Learning about what is wrong and right in your body, what the diagnosis is, what it means, what can be done about it, and what to expect in reality will give you a sense of control again. Gaining control of something small, a little at a time, will help. Getting support from other people and communicating honestly with someone about your feelings, not just about the pain, will help. Counseling with, or receiving "coaching" from a professional may be very important to gain this sense of control and lessen frustration levels. Even Muhammad Ali, Michael Jordan, and Tiger

Woods used or are using coaching.

It should be noted that the word "pain" is not on this chart. Whether the pain is lessened or not is important, but not the only important goal to work on. The levels of endurance can and need to be built up and the frustration levels can and need to be brought down whether the pain is lessened or not.

Chronic Pain Syndrome

Now let's review something called the "chronic pain syndrome." A syndrome is a complex of difficulties characterized by certain symptoms and findings. Thus, other symptoms can occur in addition to pain. Chronic usually means six months or longer. It may simply mean that which remains after healing. It seems that people can have pain syndromes without the word chronic being used; and people can have chronic pain without the full blown syndrome of issues, effects, and problems.

Let's start out with the word "pain" and also the idea of "lack of control". You are a normal person dealing fairly well with your normal life stresses, joys, and problems. Then pain enters the scene.

PAIN

What is the first feeling, besides pain, that you might experience when you hit your thumb with a hammer? What do you say or do to express this feeling?

"I feel stupid or frustrated or angry." This, or something like it, is indeed what you might feel normally, and you might express it by swearing or yelling or throwing the hammer.

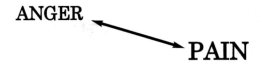

ANGER

PAIN

Anger, or feeling mad, is a normal, natural feeling that goes along with pain. Actually, it goes along with the sense of a lack of control. "I didn't control the hammer and I hit the wrong nail." Anger can be associated with a simple pain like hitting your thumb with a hammer, sitting on a tack, or stubbing your toe on the kitchen table leg. It may also go along with more long-term pain. If the pain goes away, so does the anger. However, if the pain persists, so might the anger.

Anger can make pain worse. It can make muscles tighter, making you feel more tense. How you handle anger can be important for pain management. Anger may not cause the pain, but if the pain cannot be fixed, managing anger as part of the treatment can help lessen it.

It is socially unacceptable to yell at people and punch holes in walls just because you are frustrated and angry with pain or other things that are out of your control. Yet you may let your guard down around the people you love and care about (i.e. being irritable around your family members). Consequently, you may "put a lid on anger", "bite the bullet", and "stuff it". Psychologists tell us that anger turned inward may lead to problems or even a specific problem. Do you know what this might be?

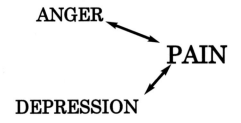

ANGER

PAIN

DEPRESSION

Anger and depression may be the most common experiences of people dealing with pain. These are very natural and understandable feelings. However, pain can feel worse when you are depressed.

You may not recognize depression. We're not talking about a disease state or a severe situation in general. However, depression can be from slight to severe and anywhere in between. There are many common symptoms which may be minor or severe or in between at any particular time. Changes in eating or sleeping patterns, problems with thinking, memory, concentration, decision making, judgment, or orientation may be experienced. You may not feel like doing anything. You may go into a room and not remember why you went there. You may forget peoples' names and phone numbers. It is like the brain is overwhelmed or divided among too many things. There are other common problems that go along with all this.

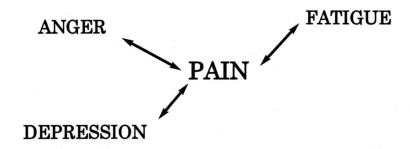

ANGER   FATIGUE

PAIN

DEPRESSION

You may simply say, "I'm just so tired all the time. I don't have any energy, no zip, I don't feel like doing anything. But I'm not depressed. What is wrong with me, doctor?".

Easy fatiguability may be a symptom of depression. Fatigue can be caused by many medical conditions: low hemoglobin, pregnancy, cancer, mononucleosis, and others . Pain can cause fatigue. Pain can wear you out. Carrying pain around is like dragging a ball and chain. And pain can be worse when you are tired.

What do you do when you get into this type of mess?

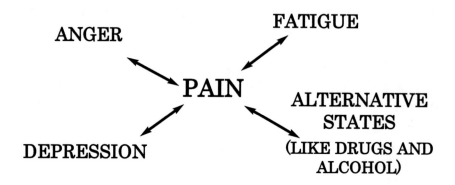

You may try to alter the whole thing. Another phrase to use is "alternative states", which implies a certain element of choice and decision-making control. You may withdraw, roll over, face the wall, turn away from everybody and everything, go to your bed room, turn the lights off, take the phone off the hook, and say "Leave me alone." You might sleep a lot. You might even think about something as drastic as suicide.

You might use drugs, alcohol, pain killers, muscle relaxants, or mood- altering medications. Pain killers prescribed for long term pain have many times caused more problems than they have helped.

There is nothing wrong with powerful analgesic medications for short-term, acute pain. There are also some pain problems that should be treated with long-term narcotic medication use, but this is not the routine. For most long-term pain problems, addicting pain killers that give only temporary relief are not the best treatment. When you use narcotic analgesics, powerful pain killers, on a long-term basis, you may have three problems: pain, dependency, and less endorphins. For long-term pain, you may need a long-term plan with less dangerous consequences. Also, the perception of pain may be worse when the effects of certain drugs or alcohol wear off.

There are many other words that can be associated with pain.

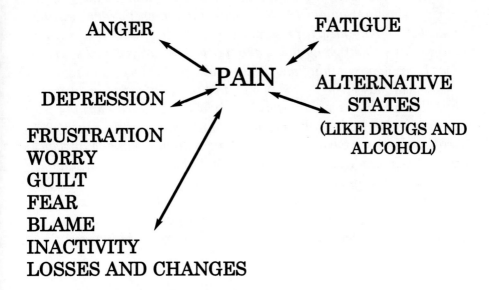

ANGER

FATIGUE

DEPRESSION

PAIN

ALTERNATIVE STATES

(LIKE DRUGS AND ALCOHOL)

FRUSTRATION
WORRY
GUILT
FEAR
BLAME
INACTIVITY
LOSSES AND CHANGES

All these other experiences can make pain worse. They can make each other worse. If you cannot make the pain go away, you can try to lessen pain by working on the various feelings and behaviors that make the pain worse.

This is the chronic pain syndrome, a whole complex of different feelings, emotions, and changes that occur with pain. These are natural feelings producing natural behaviors in attempting to deal with complex situations. How you deal with all this can be very important for there are good, appropriate, and successful ways; and there are less good, less appropriate, and less successful ways.

The pain syndrome does not always have to be associated with long term pain. The text books describe chronic pain syndrome as taking 6 months to develop. However, in reality, it seems that the syndrome can develop relatively quickly once pain occurs. The various aspects of the syndrome may snowball on you before you know it.

Patient: "*After 2 or 3 weeks of lying around, very inactive, with back and leg pain, I started to feel very irritable, on edge, angry. I barked and yelled at my 2-year-old for spilling milk in the grass. He was simply trying to help his useless-burden-on-the-family dad. I started to feel guilty, depressed, worried, more afraid. It wore me out to think about going to the bathroom. I would get tired so easily. I was doing nothing physically--no long distance running, no racquetball, no sitting at the piano, no sitting anywhere because it hurt too much. I was counting my Tylenol #3's each morning to see how many I could take each day and not run out before the next refill. I wondered what really was wrong with me emotionally; why was I such an angry person? I wasn't! I had to recognize a normal set of feelings occurring because of pain, resulting in an inability to stay active, to vent frustrations, to do things for fun and enjoyment. Once I recognized what was happening, I knew that I had to work on these feelings, not just pain, to try to improve the whole situation.*"

This is the "pain syndrome". It did not take six months to develop.

Results of the Chronic Pain Syndrome: Changes That Occur

Associated with the chronic pain syndrome are various losses or changes in a person's life. One must consider that change may not only mean loss but might also mean gain.

<u>1) Loss or change of self esteem:</u>

You might have been very strong physically, a good athlete, or a good homemaker. Your job and your position in your family may be important aspects of your self-esteem, self-concept, and self-worth. When you have the chronic pain syndrome, it becomes very difficult to keep up your position in the family and on the job.

2) Loss or change of communication:

You might quit talking with your spouse or other close persons in your life. Because you don't want to yell and bark at them or feel like a burden, you quit talking altogether. This loss of communication harms a relationship, especially marriage. Communication is improved by honestly and openly talking or writing about your feelings associated with the pain.

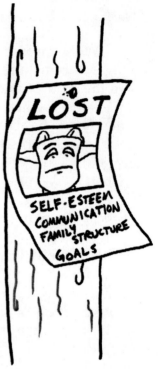

On the other hand, communication can change in a negative way. You might begin to talk only about pain. This focusing on the pain is hard on everybody involved. There was a woman who had neck pain and her spouse had heart problems. They said that in recent months these two problems were the only things they talked about. Their entire life revolved around these two medical problems. The pain and the disability may become the center and most important aspects in the affected person's life. This situation can be changed.

3) Loss or change of family structure:

You might quit playing with your children or doing other things with your family. Even simple activities such as lifting your small children to hold them may become painful experiences. You become isolated from your own family for fear of "hurting daddy's back". Family activities are done without you or with you watching from the sidelines.

4) Loss or change of goals:

With chronic pain, your whole perspective on life changes; this includes your goals. Your only goal might be to solve the pain problem. You realize that this goal could be unrealistic. You are not sure what kind of work you can do, what you will be able to do physically. Because of this uncertainty, you do not continue with life goals or develop any new goals. You feel stuck with a primary goal that is unattainable.

5) Loss or change of group support:

Your bowling team doesn't want you back anymore. Your bridge group doesn't call you anymore. You might have been a model employee on an assembly line or in construction or in a hospital or whatever for 20 years. But then with the injury and pain you are off work for a few months and then return to work on limited duty. Your fellow workers and supervisors might believe (or so you think) that you're faking it, gold-bricking. This belief is often simply due to lack of knowledge. Your friends avoid you because you feel and act irritable. You no longer hunt, fish, golf, or play cards with them anymore. Your conversation always revolves around your back problems, and your friends simply get tired of listening to you.

6) Loss or change of roles:

Roles may become reversed or at least change at home. This is sometimes referred to as power shifting. If you normally shovel the walk, cut the grass, fix the plumbing, do the housework, or laundry, and then you are injured, you may not be able to do these jobs because of pain. So your spouse, significant other, or children may have todo them. If the one with back pain was the bread winner and cannot get a job due to their pain problem, the other person may have to go to work. These role changes can cause marital conflicts and feed into the loss of self-esteem. One must find control in possibly new routines and activities. There can be power sharing in chores and tasks. It does not have to be only the loss of roles but possibly even the gain of new ones.

The results of the chronic pain syndrome need not be only losses. A better word to use might be that of "changes". You go through an identity change, such as occurs when getting married or having children. You cannot go back. You can only change and go on. A change may be for the better. A good change could occur if you work at making something positive out of the situation. For example, you might conclude, "I am gaining a certain empathy toward others with pain. I may not die of a heart attack at the age of 49 because I'm learning and practicing to deal better with stress. I have this opportunity to spend time with my children."

Friend: "My dad was laid up with a back problem one summer, and I remember it as a good summer because he was home all the time. He may not think of it as all that good, but I remember it that way."

These issues are part of the chronic pain syndrome. You may feel miserable not just because of the pain but also because of other feelings and emotions which have developed--fear, anger, depression, and other psychosocial stresses which have developed. You may also feel badly because of losses or changes in your life--self-esteem, communication, family structure, goals, group support, and roles. As you find yourself in this mess, you may need some help to get out of it, to lessen the pain as much as possible, and to live better with whatever remains.

Notes:

Chapter 6: COMMONLY ASKED QUESTIONS AND ANSWERS

Concerning Long-Term Pain

Concerning Discs

Concerning Soft Tissue Injuries, Other Conditions, And Treatment Ideas

This last chapter addresses questions posed earlier in the book more directly and specifically.

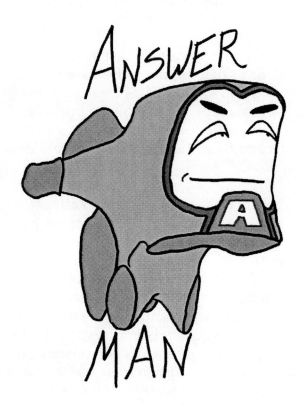

Concerning Long-Term Pain:

Are you sure he or she is not faking?
　　While there are some bad apples in every barrel, most people with long-term pain problems are not malingering or faking. There may be some functional or emotional components to a person's long-term pain problem such as fear, anger, frustration, depression, anxiety, worry, guilt, blame, or other issues. Sometimes there may even be hypochondiasis or conversion disorder or significant psychological components to a person's pain problem which increase the perception of pain or even cause the perception of pain.
　　Most of the time people are very straightforward, honest, and are struggling with medical problems that are very difficult to identify and document clearly. These medical problems may also be very difficult to treat. Chronic pain complicates the person's life in many ways. The best approach is to understand that the pain is real, not "imaginary" or psychological. The sources of the pain must be identified and explained as clearly as possible. It must be fixed if possible. If this is not possible, then at least it must be treated appropriately, to reduce the amount of pain and help the person effectively deal with the remaining pain.

If he can go to a play or do some other recreational activity, why can't he work more hours? If the person can ride a motorcycle, why can't he work?
　　Each person's medical problem is unique. Recreational activities are very important for almost everybody to help maintain mental health. Recreational activities are good for stress management. Each person's job, the physical and emotional demands and responsibilities, and each person's abilities are unique. A person may be able to perform certain recreational activities but be unable to return to a specific job that involves activities that are out-

side of certain limitations for safety and comfort. Sometimes riding a large, well-cushioned motorcycle can be much easier than a job that involves heavy lifting, standing or bending repetitively for extended lengths of time. While all of these factors have to be considered, simply because a person is trying to maintain some recreational activities, does not automatically mean that he or she can work more. Return to work depends on the specific activities and demands of the job along with specific medical limitations and restrictions.

How long does it take for things to heal? They said it would just take time but this has already been a long time.

The body begins to heal immediately after injury. Many times the injured person impairs healing by continuing self-destructive behaviors. Many times healing is not the issue. Giving pain more time "to heal" may not be the issue at times. When a problem is permanent, that means it is not going away with more time. For most injuries, healing takes place within a finite period of time, such as a few days to months. While most pain with injuries will go away in that time, in some instances the pain persists. Scar tissue around a nerve, muscles that tend to spasm easily, bone spurs that have formed and irritate sensitive structures, and many other medical problems can often cause long-term pain that will not "heal or go away" simply by giving it a little more time. If time will take care of the medical problem, fine. In other situations with long-term pain, people need to work on treatment approaches that can lessen the pain as much as possible and help deal better with whatever remains.

Why can't they just fix this problem?

Sometimes medical problems can't even clearly be diagnosed, much less fixed. Medical tests such as a CAT scan (computerized axial tomography) or MRI (magnetic resonance imaging) are done for specific reasons to answer specific questions. But tests do not show everything. A test result may be "normal" while there is a real problem, not imaginary. The diagnosis may be made based on history and examination findings.

Once the problem has been identified, it may not be possible to "fix" it. Many times fixing something, such as doing surgery for a herniated disc, can be very helpful; but also many times the risks of doing particular procedures to fix the problem outweigh the possible benefits. Many medical problems are not simple and easily fixed. Many are more complicated, hard to diagnose, hard to treat, and complicate a person's life. Problems such as chronic pain may need to be dealt with by complicated treatment approaches; not impossible, but not simple either. If it cannot be fixed, then how you manage it yourself may become extremely important.

I've been to several doctors. One tells me this, another tells me that. They can't agree and I am in between.

Such differences of opinion are often the case in trying to diagnose and treat certain medical problems. One doctor's medical opinion may differ from another physician's opinion. As in any area of life, two people looking at the same problem can view it in different ways. Also, tests can be interpreted differently. The same CAT scan films or MRI films, for example, could be read by three different radiologists with three differing results. Each person dealing with long-term pain must find a physician that he or she trusts and respects. Second opinions are fairly common and standard procedure in cases of surgery or difficult medical problems. Often the patient will need to work on treatment approaches that make sense to that person. Knowledge and assertiveness may help the injured person to be more in control. Also to look for areas of agreement or overlap in the various opinions can be helpful.

It seems that the insurance company is only out to save dollars. They don't care about me. They just force me back to work and don't care if it hurts me.

The situation may indeed be this way at times, for often the system is not fair. The people working in the system, such as claims representatives, are simply trying to do their jobs. Many times trying to save money is part of the issue.

Take control of what you can as much as you can. It will not help you to only focus on what you cannot control. It will not help you to only focus on "the way things used to be or ought to be." Learn about your medical condition, the insurance issues, your rights with respect to work issues. While the system may work very well to help you, many times it does not work so well. If you depend on the system too much to do the work, you may be very disappointed in the results. Each injured person must control, as much as possible, his or her own situation in the system concerning insurance, work, and medical issues.

Each injured person must set goals that include end points of return to employment and other life activities as appropriate within identified limitations. Return to work or other normal life activities should be done as soon as possible for the injured person's own sense of self-control. Each injured person must set very clear small steps to reach the goals. The more this type of specific goal-setting is done, the better off the person will fare within the system.

If it hurts, I am not going to do it. Pain has a purpose and it is telling me this isn't safe. At least, I don't want to be so flared-up that I can't enjoy anything after doing a particular activity.

While most pain does have a purpose, it is not always the case that pain is protective. If you have your finger in the flame of a   candle, the pain says get your finger out of there. In medicine, the diagnosis can be identified, the treatment plan can be applied as fully as possible, the person can be doing only activities that are safe, and still sometimes the pain can persist. This type of pain loses much of its "protective" purposes and becomes more or less "worthless" in terms of protecting the person.

Each injured person might have difficulty with persistent pain. It may take a while to determine your limitations. Just because it hurts doing specific activities does not mean that the activities are not safe. Often we say "if it hurts, don't do it", usually referring to particular activities that can be causing tissue damage. Many times pain can be present but not be a sign of impending tissue damage. In those cases, pushing yourself is desirable for recovery, but you don't want to push too hard. Each person, in each individual situation, needs to determine his or her own limits with guidance from the physician and rehabilitation staff.

"If it hurts, don't do it," may not apply at a particular time. You might be hurting as you are sitting still doing nothing in particular to aggravate the situation. On the other hand, the other extreme of "No pain, no gain" may not apply either. You may know full well that this approach will not work for you. It will only make things worse. You will need to find a middle ground between doing too little and doing too much. You will need to find a baseline and foundation on which you can build and gradually improve.

I can't accept that this problem is going to be permanent.
That's understandable, and you may not have to accept it at all. If the problem is relatively recent, possibly the appropriate treatment plan will make the pain go away completely. If, however, the pain has been present for a very long time, and all the appropriate treatments have been tried, then the pain may persist at a certain level indefinitely. We understand that it is difficult to believe that medical problems may be permanent.

People sometimes say, "I understand that this

problem is permanent but isn't there something that can fix it?" If you are confident that your physician has examined you and has done appropriate testing, then you need not go any further in terms of establishing a diagnosis. You may need to talk further with your physician to understand the diagnosis more clearly, to understand why further tests won't be of help, to understand why the pain lasts so long, what can and cannot be done about the pain to lessen it and live better with what remains.

The body's tissues heal in finite periods of time, but pain can persist beyond the healing phase. Scar tissue continually irritating nerve can be an example of this. While often no medical treatment can actually cure the problem, usually other approaches can lessen the pain.

A major factor here is acceptance or management of the problems. Acceptance, management of the problems, is a difficult issue and needs to be worked on daily. It does not mean giving up on any hope to lessen the pain by medical means. Medicine changes and so does each person over time. However, management and acceptance do mean a change in focus from overwhelming time and effort on medical approaches and pain focus to more focus on life and what is important in your life in spite of the pain. Management and acceptance mean coming to some kind of serenity about the fact that the problem may be permanent. But also you may need a certain willingness to only control the pain as much as possible and to make each day worthwhile in spite of the pain. Acceptance is also a process of continually moving through the various stages of grief and loss, such as anger, depression, fear, bargaining, worry, guilt, denial. Management and acceptance does not mean that you like having the pain problem, but it does mean that you are willing to do today whatever you can do to make today most profitable.

I am beginning to wonder if the problem is imaginary.

Pain is not imaginary. It is real. However, the problem causing the pain may not be due to an identifiable source on a test. Again, understand that the tests do not show everything. Pain is not imaginary and very definitely affects your emotional well-being. When you feel emotionally distraught because of the pain, you may begin to wonder whether or not being emotionally distraught is the cause of the pain. Such emotional stress contributes to the pain perception, worsening or aggravating it. Consequently, working on your own emotional well-being can help lessen pain.

If I just didn't have this pain or if they could just fix the pain problem, I wouldn't have all these other emotional, financial, relationship, vocational and recreational problems.

Most likely, this is a true statement. Sometimes, however, in reality the person did have significant life difficulties before the injury. Let us consider that the pain problem comes first and the other problems secondarily develop because of the pain. It is of interest to know that these other psychosocial problems and resulting stresses can actually worsen the pain. Pain is worse when one is depressed or more tired. Pain is worse when one is not sleeping well. Anger and anxiety tend to make muscles more tight. Therefore, working on the other problems and stresses can sometimes lessen the pain.

This person isn't doing the work he used to do, but I think he could if he wanted to. Look at the professional football quarterback who had back surgery and went back to playing professional football.

Each person's medical problem and treatment is unique. Sometimes people can return to very strenuous, sudden, jarring, jerking, twisting physical activity even after a significant back or neck surgical intervention. In other cases, however, there are significant limitations for safety and comfort after surgery. People usually want to return to their previous work or recreational activities but sometimes simply cannot because of their limitations. In our society we are very intolerant of long term problems. We think things should be fixed quick. If they are not fixed, we attribute the problem to the person; it is their own fault and weakness that keeps them injured. We must all be very careful of this attitude. It never helps the person or the situation. It probably isn't true anyway. It could be you someday dealing with a long term and not well understood problem.

I am not depressed, I am just tired all the time. I don't feel like doing anything. I have no energy, no zip. I don't know what is wrong with me.

Depression is often a difficult concept to understand. There are different kinds of depression, and varying degrees of severity. Sometimes the word "overwhelmed" is a better word to use. Often with the pain problems, people are overwhelmed by all of the effects of pain. Pain wears people out. It is like carrying around a ball and chain and never being able to set it down. You always carry it, day, night, weekends, wherever you go, you never get a rest from it. Often a certain amount of unexpressed anger, frustration, or resentments are associated with having the pain problem. People in pain are often unable to keep up their normal stress-venting or frustration-venting activities such as recreational activities or work. They have more stress and frustration on board, dealing with pain and its effects, and less ways to get rid of even normal stresses and frustrations. Feeling overwhelmed is common and it is very tiring. Things start to seem boring and it begins to take more and more energy, or so it seems, to accomplish even the simple tasks. There can be changes in sleeping patterns, changes in eating patterns, troubles with thinking, memory, concentration, judgment, orientation, decision-making, and tremendous fatigue. These and other feelings can be present to various degrees and can change from hour to hour and day to day. Such symptoms also can be seen with depression.

Why shouldn't I use pain pills? They are the only things that help. They keep me going. They make me able to keep up some normal activities.

We can kill pain with powerful narcotic drugs. We can make people unconscious. Pain-killing medications typically depress the central nervous system. They decrease the amounts of natural pain-killing chemicals (endorphins) which are actually much stronger than anything we can take or use. Each time you take a narcotic pain killer, the pain may be less for awhile. But as the pain killer wears off, your own endorphins will be lessened in amounts. The pain may actually seem worse when the pill wears off, even though the anatomy is the same. The chemistry changes. Taking pain pills can be like whipping a horse to pull a cart. It will keep going for awhile but eventually will drop, not just from pulling the cart but also from the whipping. There are some narcotic pain killers that sometimes can be used long term. Prolonged use may not be advisable because of dependency problems. These might include tolerance, increases in the amount used even though the anatomy and pain problem is not really changed, withdrawal problems, and overwhelming focus on pain medication as the main stay in treatment approaches.

If exercise makes things hurt worse, I am not going to do it. Is it really a matter of "no pain no gain"?

No, it is not a matter of "no pain no gain". Sometimes exercise can cause pain to worsen somewhat. If the exercise can be done in a very slow, gentle, gradual, consistent manner and if the person doing the exercise knows clearly that he or she is not going to be causing tissue damage, then the exercise can actually still be good in spite of causing some pain. We anticipate some pain when people start a new exercise program and use muscles, ligaments and joints that have not moved fully for a length of time. Endurance building is used to increase your own body's pain killing chemicals. A therapist or other professional might say, "If it hurts, don't do it." They may be speaking to risk of tissue damage, for example, radiating pain down the leg due to a herniated disc pushing on a nerve in the low back. The definition of "too much" pain needs to be addressed more specifically by your doctor and with you. Conditioning and endurance building exercise is usually not an all-or-none situation but rather a slow, gentle, gradual, consistent process.

Concerning Discs:

What are discs?

Discs are hockey puck-shaped cushions located in the spaces between the vertebrae (the bones). They are named by the vertebrae above and below the disc. For example, the C5-C6 disc is located between the fifth and sixth cervical (neck) vertebrae. The L4-L5 disc is located between the fourth and fifth lumbar (low back) vertebrae.

What are they made of and what do they do?

Structurally, each disc has a firm, fibrous outside layer and a liquid-like, jelly-like inner core. The outer, fibrous layer is called the annulous fibrosus. The tough fibers of the annulous fibrosus criss-cross in diagonal directions like the bands on a steel-belted radial tire. This arrangement gives the disc strength. The inner core of the disc is called the nucleus pulposus. This inside is more like liquid, grizzle, toothpaste in consistency. The nucleus pulposus made of gelatinous protein is contained by the annulous fibrosus and provides the cushion effect. Discs are the cushions or shock absorbers between the bones.

What is a "bulging" or "herniated" disc, and which is worse?

With time, wear and tear, and with injury, the outer annulous fibrosus can become damaged. This damage causes weakening of the fibrous bands resulting in a "bulging" disc. If the fibers are actually torn, the inner gelatinous core may extrude out through the annulous fibrosus, resulting in a "herniated" disc. Other terms for this condition are a "slipped", "ruptured", "protruded", "extruded" disc. Think of it like toothpaste out of a toothpaste tube. If it oozes out, we might call this "herniated or ruptured".

Better yet, think of the disc as a grape. If you squeeze a grape a little bit, it tends to bulge in the middle, as would a bulging disc. However, if you keeping applying pressure, the grape will eventually "pop." The grape covering tears and the inside of the grape shoots out, resulting in a "ruptured" or "herniated" grape. A herniated disc occurs in a similar fashion. A "contained disc" might be like the bulging grape, whereas a "non-contained disc" might be like the herniated or ruptured grape. Similarly, think of a disc like a Bismarck donut. The jelly like substance can ooze through to the outside and press against the nerve next to it, and send symptoms into an arm or leg or anyplace in the body where the nerve goes. Usually a herniated disc poses a problem only if it is pressing on a nerve root or the spinal cord.

What is "degenerated" or "deteriorated" or "dehydrated"?

If a grape (like a disc) sits on a shelf a long time and doesn't move at all, it tends to dry up, like turning into a raisin. This might be thought of as a "degenerated" or "deteriorated" or "dehydrated" disc. We all get some of this as we grow older. From the ages of twenty to the age of eighty we might lose two to six inches in height due to disc narrowing, wearing out, flattening, or drying up of the disc material (and also due to bone deterioration). This usually doesn't cause any symptoms, but certainly can cause problems if the disc herniates and irritates nearby nerves. Actually, on a percentage basis, disc disease accounts for only a small portion of pain from the spine, particularly chronic pain.

Are discs strong?

Discs are very strong. If we squeeze straight up and down on the column of bones and discs hard enough, the bones will crack and crumble before the discs will give way. However, if we squeeze with more of a slant, or wedging, the discs may "pop" or rupture. Also twisting, torque movements on the discs are very hard on them and can result in a tearing, shearing, or wearing out of the outside and a bulging through of the inside.

Can a bulging disc become a herniated disc?

Yes. A disc can heal in the wrong shape and still be strong, but it can also be weakened and at risk of herniating.

What can X-rays show?

We can see vertebrae but not discs on simple x-rays of the back or neck. X-rays may help rule out other pathology, such as fractures, tumors, etc. The x-rays go right through a disc. Discs are shown only by CT or MRI scanning. Usually problems can be seen, but indeed may not show well. However, if a disc is worn or herniated, that disc space may be narrowed because of the lessened volume of the nucleus pulposus. So, if we see a narrow disc space on regular x-rays, this finding may or may not suggest significant disc disease or pathology at that level.

My CT scan showed a deteriorated and bulging disc, but my doctor said this was "normal". How can this be "normal"? I'm hurting like crazy?

Often people may have these findings without any symptoms at all. Aging is normal. The older we are, the more "pathology" is seen. And what is seen may or may not be significant, may or may not be the cause of the symptoms. Many people without symptoms of pain have bulging, deteriorated, or even herniated discs as seen on CT or MRI scans. The doctor has to put the history, the physical examination findings, and test results all together and decide what he or she truly thinks is the cause of the specific symptoms.

What is "spurring"? And what about "arthritis"?

When a disc is narrowed, or worn out, or bulged, or herniated, or "flattened out like a pancake", the body may form calcium, bone spurring, "osteophytic spurring", all around the edges of the bones above and below the disc in an attempt to hold the disc still, to protect it. This may take months or years to form. It may not cause any symptoms. However, if it is next to a nerve and irritating the nerve, it certainly can cause symptoms. The word "arthritis" is sometimes overused. However, "osteoarthritis" or "spondylosis" is the name given to the bony spurring seen around the spine and joints of the spine.

Can scar tissue form, and can it be helpful or harmful?

Scar tissue can form around a herniated or bulging disc to help strengthen and support the disc. Scar tissue can help the discs be strong even after they have been injured. However, the discs can continue to bulge more and more, and therefore, a person with disc pathology may have to be careful with activities, not to damage the disc further. Scar tissue that forms after surgery may irritate near by nerves, and cause symptoms of pain or numbness or tingling, etc.

Can a disc go back to its normal shape given enough time, and can a disc heal in the wrong shape and still cause pain?

The toothpaste can go back into the toothpaste tube if it wasn't out very far in the first place. There is a lot of debate about what effect various treatments really have on the discs (traction, chiropractic manipulation). Discs can heal in the wrong shape and still cause pain.

Sometimes the pain goes away or lessens for a while, but then comes back again. Why is this?

The disc is dynamic, changing its shape and position somewhat with movement. The nerve next to the disc only has so much room. If the nerve is irritated by the disc during or after certain movements, such as twisting, bending, or lifting, then the nerve may become swollen. This leads to more irritation which in turn leads to more swelling, etc. This can come and go, and should be watched closely for any signs of progressive nerve damage.

Can they replace the inside of the disc with something else?

After surgery to remove a disc, the body often forms fibrous, hard, calcified scar tissue, inside and around the operated part of the disc. The disc space, however, can be narrowed after surgery and result in joint problems, nerve irritation, continued symptoms into a limb. Fusion surgery, using other bone or metal to hold the vertebrae solidly together, might be done sometimes, and indeed might keep the vertebrae apart enough to prevent the nerves from being compressed.

Can they operate on the same disc more than once?

Yes. At the first operation they may only take the loose nucleus pulposus material, or the material that comes out easily (like removing from the assembly line only the person who is not doing his job). Sometimes the remaining material can bulge or herniate later and the person may need another operation.

I don't want to know about this stuff. I just want it fixed so I can go back to work again.

This is understandable. However, once a disc is damaged, it may not be the same as it was before the injury, no matter what is done to help. The person may have to return to work with certain limitations for safety and comfort. Other things can be done to take pressure off an injured disc, such as weight loss, and good posture and body mechanics. Also, a good exercise program can help keep the surrounding structures as healthy as possible.

Why don't they just do a CT scan or better yet an MRI and just find out what the problem is and fix it?

Things aren't this easy or simple. The doctor orders tests usually when looking for something specific. It is not that one test is better than another, rather it is that the doctor orders the test that best helps rule out or in certain pathologic processes that may be suspected. If what is suspected to be the problem will not show on a particular test, then that test will most likely not be ordered.

The doctors have to be concerned about a possible disc problem before they will order tests that might show discs. They have to be concerned about spinal cord, joint or bone problems before ordering tests that show these structures. Often the test results are "normal" even though the doctor knows there is something wrong. The tests don't show everything.

This is part of why it is difficult to "just fix the problem". Often the problem does not even show up clearly on the tests. It is hard to "just fix" something you can't even see clearly. Back and neck problems, particularly if chronic, usually are not "fixable" with surgery. This is why it is important that the various conservative (active and passive) measures be carried out to give you the best comfort level possible, to lessen pain as much as possible, and to help you to live better with whatever remains.

Concerning Soft Tissue Injuries, Other Conditions, And Treatment Ideas:

What do they mean by soft tissue injury, myofascial pain, muscle ligament strain, musculoskeletal pain?

Soft tissue injury refers to damage to the ligaments, tendons, fascia and muscles. This sometimes might be called "musculoligamentous strain" or "myofascial pain". "Myo" refers to muscle and "fascial" refers to the connective tissue or bands of tissue that surround the bundles of muscle fibers. Most acute and chronic neck and back pain is due to injuries to these structures. For example, neck pain following a "whiplash" injury (sudden acceleration-deceleration injury) during a rear-end collision may be the result of soft tissue injury. Such an injury causes a localized irritation from tearing and stretching in ligaments and muscle fibers. This may include the ligaments surrounding the facet joints in the neck or back. This irritation sets up a reflex muscle spasm. The natural response of the body to such irritation is to guard and protect itself by holding that body part (i.e. neck) still by means of muscle tightness, spasm, or contraction. This muscle contraction further aggravates the pain, resulting in more spasm and pain. Muscle tightness hurts if it last too long. Tight muscles tend to get tired. Tired muscles tend to get tight. You can see that the proverbial vicious circle develops with pain-spasm-pain-spasm-etc.

Are they sure something isn't being missed? I mean I hurt soft tissue and pulled muscles before but that pain went away in a few days or weeks. This pain isn't going away.

It is possible that something is being missed. Tests don't show everything. You need to talk with your doctor about your specific questions concerning his or her reasons and opinions for the diagnosis that has been made or is being used at this time. The diagnosis is made on the basis of your history (the specific information about your symptoms and what happened to you), the physical examination, and the diagnostic testing. Even though the results of diagnostic tests may be "normal", this does not mean that the problem is psychological (although it could be so). Just because the tests are normal does not mean there is not a physical reason for the pain or that something is being missed. Again, tests don't show everything.

Each diagnostic procedure is performed specifically to evaluate certain anatomical, chemical or physiological functions to determine the cause of the pain. For example, simple x-rays basically show bones. The CT (computerized tomographic) scan shows both bone and soft tissue, but not completely. A myelogram is another anatomical test which provides a different perspective of back and neck problems but it still does not reveal everything. The same is true of the MRI (magnetic resonance imaging), which shows significant anatomical detail. Electromyography (EMG) and thermography show the function of nerves but can also come back "normal" even in the face of severe pain.

Normal test results do not mean that you are not in pain or that the problem is imaginary or something is being missed. Normal tests indicate that certain causes for pain which were evaluated were not found to be present. But there may be something else causing the pain that does not show up well on tests and needs to be discussed with you in detail for your own understanding. Even though the tests may be normal, you still need detailed information about what is going on, what can be done about it, and what to expect for the future.

What are trigger points? Why would I want to have injections in these areas that are sore?
A trigger point is a hyperirritable (very sensitive) spot within a taut band of a skeletal muscle that is painful on compression and can give rise to characteristic referred

pain, tenderness, and autonomic phenomena such as local temperature increases, sweating, and numbness. Trigger points can be active (pain and tightness) or latent (tightness only). Trigger points are localized areas where the muscle contracts so much that it may cause a knot that you can actually feel under the skin.

These painful areas can persist for a long time - sometimes years - and are usually not easily treated by conventional forms of physical therapy. A trigger point is like having a "charlie horse" in that area of muscle that just doesn't go away. The trigger point serves as a source of pain, resulting in reflex muscle spasm by the surrounding muscle fibers with increased body activity. They can also become very painful when the person is inactive to long or maintains one position for extended lengths of time.

Typically, when the doctor is examining you, deep pressure in the region of a trigger point can cause such pain in that area that it causes you to wince, resulting in the "positive jump sign." Sometimes pain as well as tingling sensation can extend down an arm or leg from the trigger point, a phenomenon called referred pain.

Trigger point injections may be quite useful in the treatment program. Often 1% Xylocaine is used because of its safety and availability. A small amount is used, approximately 0.5 to 1 cc of the 1% Xylocaine solution. The trigger point is injected and the needle is directed in a circular pattern around the trigger point. Xylocaine has a vasodilatory effect on the trigger point increasing capillary circulation. It also has a curarae-like action on the myofilaments (very small fibers of muscle). This relaxes the taut band and releases the physiologic contracture within the muscle.

Patients often ask if cortisone is used. Typically it is not used. Research has not shown that there is significant inflammation or swelling in the muscle or trigger points. Therefore, cortisone, which lessens inflammation, is usually not necessary.

Following the trigger point injection, the taut band may be more supple and trigger points may no longer refer pain. You may not want or need trigger point injections. Your doctor may not feel they would be appropriate in your situation. You may want to discuss this in more detail with your doctor.

What is carpal tunnel syndrome? What can I expect for the future?

Another example of nerve pressure which may cause neck pain, but usually does not, is carpal tunnel syndrome. In this condition, the median nerve as it runs through the middle front of the wrist may be compressed within the wrist. Typically carpal tunnel syndrome causes numbness, tingling, and pain into the thumb, index and middle fingers which awaken the person at night or occur while using the hands or driving. Weakness in the distribution of the median nerve can also occur. Pain in this situation can be referred into the arm, shoulder or neck.

There are actually three main nerves that go into the hand from the arm: radial (to the thumb), median (to part of the thumb, the index, third and part of the fourth fingers), and ulnar (to the fifth and part of the fourth digits). The median nerve goes through a tunnel of connective tissue in the middle of the front part of your wrist (carpal area). Sometimes the tunnel can become narrowed, for various reasons, and pinch or damage the median nerve. If the problem is present, it should be observed closely by your physician, watching for any progressive nerve damage. Clinical examination and EMG (electromyogram, a nerve test with pins put into the and which measures the speed and quality of electricity traveling along the nerves and into the muscles) can help in this monitoring process. Discontinuing the excessive overuse or misuse or trauma of the wrist and median nerve can be part of the treatment plan, and if needed, surgical intervention can be accomplished.

The problem might worsen, improve, or simply cause you symptoms off and on through your life. Some have experienced the symptoms for decades without any obvious progressive difficulties. Some may have significant progression of nerve damage and resultant muscle deterioration and worsening of painful symptoms. You need to discuss this issues specifically with your doctor, because each individual person and situation is different.

What is thoracic outlet syndrome? What can I expect for the future?

Pressure on nerves in the shoulder or arm can cause referred pain into the neck and down into the arm and even into the hand. A fairly common problem in this category as a consequence of injury is thoracic outlet syndrome. With this condition, pressure from muscle spasm, cervical rib, fibrous bands of tissue and even scar tissue from injury and other causes can irritate the nerves in the brachial plexus. In addition to neck pain, typical symptoms include numbness and tingling along the inside of the forearm and hand and into the ring and little fingers. Cold, burning, prickly pins and needles sensations and weakness can occur. Raising arms into the air as in combing or brushing the hair or painting a ceiling may increase these symptoms.

People who sleep with their arms over their heads are at risk for development of symptoms, but house painters, hairdressers, and truck drivers also may develop problems because of the position of their arms above the shoulders. The condition may also occur due to muscle tightness around the area after neck or upper back trauma.

Treatment consists of conservative measures such as physical therapy and stretching exercises, or surgical removal of the first or top rib or congenital rib. Conservative measures are effective 70 percent of the time.

The problem might worsen, improve, or simply cause you to experience symptoms off and on through your life. You need to discuss this question specifically with your doctor, because each individual person and situation is different.

What is mechanical back or neck pain? What are facet joints?

Mechanical low back pain results from irritation to the movable joints in the low back area such as the facets and sacroiliac joints. The vertebrae connect with one another by joints, termed facets. The facets allow movement in both front-to-back and side-to-side directions. Each vertebra has four facets. Two facets pivot on the vertebra sitting on top and two facets pivot on the vertebra below. The facets provide flexibility of movement for the vertebral column, permitting one to bend in all directions. Like all joints of the body such as the shoulders and knuckles, the facets are lined with tissue and surrounded by a thin capsule of ligament tissue which is pain-sensitive. And, like these joints, the facets may become irritated and painful producing spine pain. The facet joints are at every level, on both sides, up and down the neck and back.

Mechanical pain can be present in the neck and back resulting from irritation of the joints there as well. This type of pain comes and goes. With rest there is little or no pain. With movement such as bending forward and back or side to side, the pain becomes prominent into the neck or back areas, usually in the middle but spreading in fairly diffuse patterns. Neither pain or other sensations such as numbness or tingling course very far down the arms or legs. Often joint problems in the back send symptoms down into the buttock or thighs but not so much below the knees. Joint problems in the neck send symptoms across the shoulders, around the back of the neck, in various patterns depending on which joints are involved. The symptoms are diffuse rather than specifically localized to particular nerve root patterns.

Facet joint problems also may result in pain when extending the spine or bending backwards. The person may have difficulty lying prone or on the abdomen because of the back extension. The person may have difficulty bending over the sink to shave, brush teeth, wash dishes because the joints are being held in an uncomfortable position for too long. Bending forward to pick   something up off the floor might be easy, but getting back up from that position may be very difficult. Extending the head and neck such as looking up to the sky or into a high cupboard may hurt the neck.

What is fibromyalgia? What can I expect for the future?

Fibromyalgia, a term often used to describe a disorder with similar symptoms to myofascial pain syndrome. However, with myofascial pain syndrome, trauma usually precedes the muscle involvement, and the symptoms are relatively localized to the area of involvement. With fibromyalgia there is usually no trauma and the symptoms are usually much more diffuse throughout the body. Tender spots of fibromyalgia are most often found at the insertion of muscle into bone, whereas trigger points of myofascial pain can be felt in the bulk of the muscle. The key is that myofascial pain is a regional pain whereas fibromyalgia is widespread.

The criteria for fibromyalgia include major and minor clinical findings: *next page...*

Major clinical criteria:
 1. *Chronic, generalized aches, pains, or stiffness: axial, upper, lower, bilateral parts of body.*
 2. *Multiple tender points at characteristic locations: at least 11 of the following 18 bilateral areas: Occiput, Lower cervical, Trapezius, Supraspinatus, Second rib, Lateral epicondyle, Gluteal, Greater trochanter, Knees.*
 3. *Absence of other systemic condition to account for these symptoms.*

Other clinical criteria:
 1. *Disturbed sleep (morning fatigue and stiffness)*
 2. *Generalized fatigue and tiredness*
 3. *Subjective swelling and numbness*
 4. *Pain in neck and shoulders*
 5. *Chronic headaches*
 6. *Irritable bowel syndrome*
 7. *Deconditioning*

Fibromyalgia is probably more common than is understood, and may not really be a single discrete condition. "Myo" refers to muscle, "fibro" refers to the fibers in the muscle, "algia" means pain.

No one is sure about the specific relationship to other medical conditions such as rheumatoid arthritis. However, fibromyalgia may be an initial manifestation of hypothyroidism. It may also be related to viral illnesses, hepatitis, mononucleosis, and a fairly common heart condition called mitral valve prolapse (MVP). Some research has demonstrated elevated levels of substance-P, a neurotransmitter, in the spinal fluid. Other research has shown lowered levels of a particular growth hormone in the spinal fluid. Fibromyalgia is not routinely diagnosed and the average duration of symptoms at the time of diagnosis may be 5 years.

Treatment may include non-steroidal antiinflammatory drugs, tricyclic antidepressants or other types of antidepressants, muscle relaxants, physical therapy, relaxation techniques, stress management techniques, and exercise programs. All may work to relieve some of the symptoms such as local pain, stiffness, and sleep difficulties. Steroids do not really work for this condition.

What is reflex sympathetic dystrophy? What can I expect for the future? Will I damage anything if I use the limb too much? What is too much?
Reflex sympathetic dystrophy is a diagnosis or condition that involves abnormal responses of the nerves and blood vessels of the body. It is sometimes called "complex regional pain syndrome" or "sympathetically maintained pain". It is like a "short-circuiting" of the part of the nervous system which is not normally under conscious control. This is the "autonomic nervous system" which takes care of things "automatically".

The sympathetic nervous system, a part of the autonomic nervous system, is responsible for regulating bodily functions such as the temperature and circulation of the extremities, blood pressure, muscle tightness, sweating, and many other functions. The sympathetic nervous system is "in sympathy" with the environment. If you cut your hand, the blood vessels respond by constricting in order to help stop the bleeding. It may or may not work depending at least in part on how bad the cut is. If somehow, the sympathetic nervous system "thinks" you are cut, and in reality you are not cut, the blood vessels may still constrict. This might result in pain, numbness, tingling, cold, blue color in the area affected.

The sympathetic nervous system role in the maintenance of blood flow to the skin and muscles of the limbs is where our interest is focused. Due to a major or minor trauma, the sympathetic network may become hyper-excited. If it does, the network responds with a reflex vasoconstriction of small arteries in the extremity. This response is not a problem unless the sympathetic receptors don't return to their normal state, allowing for passive vasodilation and adequate blood perfusion to the area. Excessive voluntary guarding or holding the extremity stiff and still too much may also contribute to worsening of the condition.

The short-circuiting of the sympathetic nervous system or the continual hyper-excitement of the sympathetic receptors results in symptoms of pain, temperature changes (usually cold), sweating, abnormal hair and nail growth, and ultimately atrophy of the muscles from disuse. Even though the limb may be cold, the pain may be described as burning or stabbing. The decreased blood flow results in decreased oxygen delivery to the area. The skin may be mottled. The temperature may be decreased. Waste products build up because of the lessened circulation. Fluid retention may occur in the limb. The person may be hypersensitive to touch in the area and exhibit avoidance behavior. There may be poor response to conventional TENS (transcutaneous electrical nerve stimulator); it may actually aggravate the pain.

This condition is estimated to be a problem in 10-20% of all people dealing with chronic long-term pain. This equates to 6-12 million people in this country. It is not a rare occurrence. The diagnosis is made by the physician at the time of the examination. The problem may be misdiagnosed since it can be a multi-symptom/multi-syndrome disease. Thermography may be the only diagnostic tool available to better define subtle changes in temperature not otherwise seen objectively. Bone scan might also be helpful in objectively noting changes in bone usually later on in the disease process. The condition does not always progress or worsen, however.

The most effective treatment for this disorder is medication to stabilize the circulation. Sympathetic nerve blocks can be helpful in the diagnosis and treatment of RSD. Sometimes surgery to destroy the sympathetic nerve into the painful area is necessary. Treatment needs to focus on the return of the sympathetic receptors to normal tonic activity; in other words, they need to slow down. Normally electrical activity travels through little nerves to the blood vessels and results in normal vasomotor tone. This is the tone of the little muscles in the walls of the blood vessels. This controls the constriction and dilitation of the blood vessels. The electricity travels at a rate of about 1-8 pulses per second. If the pulses travel faster, at about 30 pulses per second, full activation (i.e. vasoconstriction) occurs. This seems to be part of the problem. When the nerves are irritated, the electrical pulses are too fast. A particular TENS unit, Spectrum Max-SD, stimulates sympathetic receptors with a pulse rate more like their own normal signal. This unique pulse aids in slowing hyperactive receptors and breaking reflex vasoconstriction to return to normal vasomotor tone.

A person dealing with this condition must use the body part or limb in order to prevent disuse atrophy and bone deterioration. You most likely will not damage anything if you use the limb too much. It is impossible to say what is "too much" in general. Each person is different. However, if you use the limb too little, bone deterioration (osteoporosis) can gradually occur.

What about diet and pain control?

Dietary and nutritional information is often controversial, unclear, and unproved scientifically. However, some very good ideas, all of which have some basis in fact are presented. At least four obvious ways in which nutrition and eating habits can influence the health of your back, including the spinal column and its supporting muscles and connective tissues are: *1. Your weight (ideal versus overweight). 2. Vitamins, minerals, and nutrients which are necessary to build and maintain strong bones and connective tissues. 3. Excessive consumption of sugar and/or animal protein which can rob the body and bones of vital nutrients. 4. General physical health and stamina.*

Let's examine these areas in more detail. Overweight often leads to poor posture, both of which cause excessive strain on the vertebrae and supporting tissues. This strain can contribute to muscle fatigue. The excess load of body weight the back must support can easily pull the vertebrae out of alignment when doing very little activity. This, of course, can be worse when the body is subjected to a stress such as lifting, pulling or twisting. A healthy back in good condition should more easily be able to withstand the stresses of daily movements as long as the movements are not excessive. When one's back has already suffered a strain or injury, such as from an accident, any overweight or poor posture places an additional burden on already tender and weakened back structures. Eating out of boredom is one of the primary reasons for compulsive eating, poor nutrition and overweight. Many people use food as a crutch to protect themselves from emotional or physical pain--a way to "forget" for a while.

Another cause of overweight is nutritional deficiencies due to consumption of refined, denatured foods, which disrupt the appetite mechanism, resulting in overeating. The body craves the nutrients which it lacks to function properly and this signal is misinterpreted as hunger and food cravings. Eating a proper balance of whole foods containing all the necessary nutritional elements will help to normalize the appetite. An adequate intake of certain vitamins, minerals, and nutrients are necessary to build and maintain strong bones and healthy connective tissue structures. Calcium, magnesium, and phosphorous must be supplied in the proper balance together with vitamin D which aids in the assimilation and use of these minerals in the body. When too little calcium is supplied, minerals are withdrawn from bones, causing decalcification, and porous and fragile bones. A calcium deficiency can also lead to nervousness and muscle cramps and spasms. Lack of magnesium can cause muscle weakness.

Some back problems are caused by disintegration and weakening of the vertebrae and connective tissue of the back. Vitamin C is essential to the formation of collagen, which holds body cells together and is concentrated in connective tissue, cartilage, and body ligaments. This vitamin can help rebuild these tissues to increase back strength and allow a return to a more active life. Adequate calcium is also necessary to help in the formation of collagen.

A lack of vitamin E can cause weak muscles and poor posture, leading to pressure on the nerves of the back, and back pain. Bone porosity and calcium migration to deposits in the soft tissues ("bone spurs") can also result from a vitamin E deficiency. An adequate intake of vitamin E also increases physical endurance due to more efficient oxygenation of body tissues. Other nutrients which are especially important for the health of the back include manganese and adequate dietary protein. Excessive sugar consumption distorts the calcium-phosphorous relationship in the blood, causing a calcium imbalance. This may result in brittle and easily fractured bones. An overconsumption of meat robs the body of calcium, magnesium, niacin and vitamin B6. Beef, which contains 25 times as much phosphorous as calcium, can cause calcium and magnesium deficiencies. Processed, refined and denatured foods also rob the body of vital nutrients. Emphasis on eating mineral-rich "whole" foods will provide these necessary food elements.

Besides these specific factors, proper nutrition is essential to promote general health, improve body strength, and increase endurance and resistance to disease.

How can exercise help my problems?

Think of any fun way that you enjoy moving your body--and that, believe it or not, is exercise! When you do that enthusiastically, it becomes not a chore, but fun! You may not be able to move as you did before you were hurt, but you need to move slowly, gently, gradually. As you work on "cross training", doing something gently like walk or walk in water, or nautilus, or gentle exercises with your arms or legs, you may eventually be more able to do what you really want to without causing significant flare-ups of pain. To many people, exercise means calisthenics (one-two-three-four), jogging (puff, pant), or some equally impossible (worse than work!) activity. So some people like to jog-- that's fine, but it's not for everyone. Each person's body is different in its exercise needs, abilities and physical condition. If you don't regularly exercise strenuously, you should start slowly, avoid excess strain and build up gradually to greater activity levels. If you are older, or have certain medical conditions such as heart disease or back/neck strain, it's important to check with your doctor and start slowly, gently, gradually.

Exercise is so closely connected with diet that it can almost be considered a nutrient. Walking invigorates, clears the head, fills the lungs with fresh air, and stimulates blood circulation. But again start slowly and gradually. You don't have to walk fast to make gains. Exercise also helps to restore the body's natural appetite regulating system. It is estimated that 40% of Americans are overweight. Two major causes include overeating (or improper eating) and inactivity. Since the body mechanism which adjusts appetite to energy needs is regulated by physical activity, sedentary living causes the appetite to go out of control. If you are reasonably active, it is much easier to keep your appetite in line with what your body actually needs. So try to take a walk or other exercise daily--the calories burned increase with the intensity of the exercise. A sensible exercise program will actually reduce appetite while it increases energy, especially if done before a meal. By balancing exercise with moderate eating, you can maintain your ideal weight throughout life.

Other beneficial effects of exercise are that it promotes flexibility and endurance, strengthens and develops the cardiovascular system and the ability of the body to utilize oxygen efficiently, and helps you feel better and more relaxed without tiring as easily.

Exercise can be as natural as increasing your daily activity, or spending more time doing an activity with a higher level of energy consumption. It should be easy enough and enjoyable enough to make a lifetime commitment, yet strenuous enough to derive maximum physical benefit from the activity. One cannot emphasize enough, however, the importance of starting out very slowly, gently, gradually, consistently, and building up over a sufficient amount of time. This is probably true for anyone, but certainly true for someone with back or neck or other pain problems.

Be sure to stretch your muscles before exercise, and gradually slow down after, to prevent muscle injury and to allow the heart to gradually adjust its pace without abrupt changes.

What are some possible exercise options? Fun activities that are good for you include: biking, running, swimming, dancing, skiing, yoga, tennis, canoeing, skating, walking, nautilus, tai-chi, low impact aerobics, water aerobic exercises. You might have liked running long distance and never really liked walking. However, walking with your child along with you can be a new and enjoyable experience. Maybe you liked playing softball but cannot do it now like you used to. Maybe being the umpire is an alternative. At least you would be in charge of something again. These ideas may seem inappropriate for you in your own situation. They may not seem fun like things were before you were hurt. But you have to think of something for yourself. Make your own list of what YOU like to do--then begin!

You might lose weight if desired. You might increase endorphins and lessen pain eventually. You might increase endurance and be able to do more physically and not cause a giant flare-up of pain after the activity. But the best reason of all to exercise is--you'll look and feel better!

Notes:

It Is In Your Head

Dr. Ralph McKinney, my friend and mentor, once wrote an article titled "It Is In Your Head". Learn what he was referring to as you read the article below. It is included here courtesy of Dr. McKinney.

After many years of working with people and chronic pain, and advising them that "It's not in your head," I have decided that I am wrong. However, patients have pain in various portions of their bodies as a result of a variety of diseases and mishaps. Medical tests (of the body) often show no physical cause, or point to a cause which is so minute that it could not possibly cause the great discomfort experienced by the patient. Conversely, we know of many people who have very abnormal medical test findings, but no symptoms to accompany the abnormality.

While testing may be fairly negative for findings, patients often receive a smorgasbord of treatments ranging from physical therapy to exercise to injections, etc. Such treatments may have poor or time-limited outcomes. Are treatments so bad and medicines so ineffective that they produce no results? If surgery is the only "real answer," why are doctors so reluctant to recommend it until all else has failed?

Over the years, we have treated thousands of patients with chronic pain. They frequently were hurt in motor vehicle accidents or Worker's Compensation incidents. While these patients differ widely in age, education, employment, and other demographic features, they shared certain commonalties. They were generally friendly, nurturing people who took on a <u>great deal</u> of responsibility. They were often the people with several jobs who managed the household with small children or had similar circumstances. They were frequently abused as children or in marriages; had taken adult responsibility as children; did not shrink from challenges; were under a good deal of stress currently and for the ear before injury; and tended to be perfectionistic and demanding of themselves. The individuals with Worker's Compensation injuries usually did not like some important aspect of their job while those injured in motor vehicle accidents were <u>almost always</u> the "hittees." I often wonder if the "hitters" did not get injured or went elsewhere for their treatment. Many of our patients were dissatisfied with some important aspect of life and often felt a lack of social support from those around them. The question occurs to me, "why should injured people have <u>any</u> commonality much less so many features in common?" One last feature is key in answering this question. These people, with so many sources of stress and so many reasons to be angry, frightened, or overwhelmed, tended to keep painful emotions to themselves for a variety of reasons. "Nobody wants to hear about it." "Nobody would understand." "What's the use of complaining?" "I don't feel like a man talking about my feelings." Etcetera. They had good reasons for keeping emotions to themselves and had learned the skill in difficult periods of their past. But "not talking about it," which kept a child out of trouble many years ago, only adds fuel to the fire of the adult who is suffering today.

When a person has physical or emotional stresses, they begin to feel these stresses deeply and personally. When they decide not to express them, then the energy that is the emotion goes directly to the painful site and increases the pain. It is as though the body is your good friend who serves you unselfishly. When the body tells you of it's concerns (i.e., pain), you respond to your friend saying, "I'm not interested," adding insult to injury. The same would be true with emotional upsets which frequently accompany injury. Equipped with emotions to produce guidance and direction, such individuals may ignore the guidance and suppress the emotions, increasing their pain. Why would they do this?

What we now know is that anger, fear, sadness, and other emotions are natural sources of guidance. If suppressed, they increase stress symptoms including pains, sleeplessness, concentration and memory problems. If useful and productive expression of emotion is undertaken, then stress symptoms are reduced and pain relieved. This is true whether the uncomfortable emotion is attached to current events or those far distant in time, or whether related to pain conditions per se or not. Many studies have validated these statements and research has demonstrated significant improvement in a wide variety of conditions such as asthma, cancer, and arthritis by the simple act of writing about upsetting situations in one's life. There are specific rapid ways of developing a coping style in which one can let go of the stresses that support poor health and use the emotions that put you in charge of your life. Your psychologist could help you in learning how. Many people feel that using the assistance of a psychologist is an unnecessary crutch in life. However, if Mohamed Ali and Michael Jordan could use a coach to become successful in their endeavors, why shouldn't you? A coach can help you focus properly and sharpen your skills. The ability to handle it? "It's all in your head!"

About the author:

Jay F. Tracy, PA-C, Psy.D., L.P. is a physician assistant and clinical psychologist. He is also an RN, registered nurse, and CCM, certified case manager. He was co-director of Rehabilitation Associates, Back and Neck Rehabilitation and Pain Management Program at The Minneapolis Clinic of Neurology, Ltd. in Minneapolis, Minnesota. He worked at this clinic from 1975 through 2001. He has also worked in the Department of Neurosurgery at the Veterans Administration Hospital in Minneapolis. He completed his doctorate in clinical psychology in 2000. His internship was at the Chronic Pain Program at Sister Kenny Institute at Abbott Northwestern Hospital, Minneapolis, Minnesota. This is where he has continued working since mid 2001. He has worked closely with physicians, psychologists, nurses, physical therapists, exercise physiologists, vocational counselors, and various other allied health personnel in caring for patients dealing with pain and other neurologic problems. He has authored many articles and lectured widely on these topics.

ISBN 1553694155-5

9 781553 694151